Other books

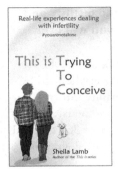

Infertility sucks doesn't it? You shouldn't feel alone whilst on your journey to having a baby. Read real-life experiences and thoughts from the fabulous TTC community, who want to support you and let you know that #youarenotalone. Available in print and as an ebook.

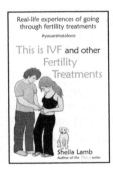

Have you recently found out you'll need IVF, or another fertility treatment to get pregnant? It's worrying and scary isn't it? Read these short stories and real-life experiences - of what to expect emotionally - from infertility warriors. All your feelings are normal and you will survive with our support.
Available in print and as an ebook.

Real-life experiences of the dreaded two-week wait
#youarenotalone

This is the Two Week Wait

Sheila Lamb
Author of the *This is* series

Are you about to go through the dreaded two-week wait? Whether this is your first or you've been here before, this wait has to be one of the hardest times on the journey to becoming a parent.
Available in print and as an ebook.

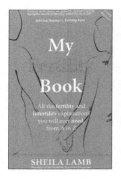

My Fertility Book; All the fertility and infertility explanations you will ever need, from A to Z

Are you stressed navigating the world of conception? Do you feel overwhelmed by the sheer amount of infertility information available online? This comprehensive, jargon-free book explains over 200 medical and non-medical terms. Available in print and as an ebook.

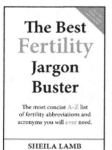

FREE EBOOK

Feeling overwhelmed by the infertility language? Confused with what the abbreviations and acronyms stand for on social media, Facebook groups and websites? All is made clear in this invaluable resource. Available as a FREE ebook – download from www.mfsbooks.co.uk

Real-life experiences from the
baby loss community
#youarenotalone

This is
Pregnancy
and Baby Loss

Sheila Lamb
Author of the *This is* series

IMPORTANT NOTICE

You may have noticed that the title of this book includes the term 'pregnancy loss'; many people will be more familiar with the term 'miscarriage'. However, I looked up the origin of the word and read that it was over 400 years old and that it meant 'mistake, error, failure', and from the 17th century – 'the fatal expulsion of a foetus from the womb before term.' You may argue that these words are the right ones to use, but for a woman and her partner who have experienced the loss of a baby during pregnancy, regardless as to whether she was five or fifteen weeks pregnant, they are hurtful, suggest she's to blame or that there is something wrong with her. Bear in mind that a pregnancy loss can occur due to issues with the egg, sperm or womb. So, after posting on Instagram my findings and asking for other people's thoughts on the word 'miscarriage', there was a unanimous agreement that using the word in the 21st Century, gives the wrong impression of the suffering and trauma associated with a pregnancy loss. Therefore, all the pregnancy loss contributors wanted to only use the words 'pregnancy loss' in their contribution. However, on occasion I have left the word 'miscarriage' in, because it's in the contributors' social media information, it's what the medical profession use, or it lends itself to their story. But my hope for the future is that nobody will use or hear the word.

Published in 2020 by MFSBooks.com

Copyright © Sheila Lamb 2020

Cover Illustration Sheila Alexander

Cover Design Marketing Hand

Copy Editor Sherron Mayes, The Editing Den

Illustrations Phillip Reed

Print ISBN 978-1-9993035-5-6

A CIP catalogue record for this book is available from the British Library.

Dedicated to every Mamma, Daddy and baby who are not together on Earth

Disclaimer

This book is intended purely to share people's real-life experiences of pregnancy loss, ectopic pregnancy and baby loss, offering words of support and comfort. It is written in their words; their experience is not medical advice. It does not replace the advice and information from your healthcare specialist, such as your doctor, nurse or other health expert. Nor is it a substitute for counselling or coaching. The author does not accept liability for readers who choose to self-prescribe. If brand names are mentioned, the author does not endorse the product or company.

The information provided must not be used for diagnosing or treating a health problem or disease.

This information was correct at the time of publication and has been interpreted by the author.

Foreword

Everyone has heard of 'miscarriage' and baby loss. Many people know how common it is and have even experienced it themselves. Yet, for some reason, it remains a subject still shrouded in secrecy. One of the things that is so important about Sheila Lamb's book is by bringing multiple voices together in one place, she uncovers the lived and shared experience of so many. In doing this she has created a place where compassion is nurtured and nourished.

As someone who has written and spoken publicly about my own experience of pregnancy loss, one of the things that struck me as soon as I was open was that people started to say: 'That happened to me and I feel that too.' There is huge comfort in this.

Within these pages you will find stories of first trimester loss; full term still birth; ectopic pregnancy; recurrent pregnancy loss and more. If you are someone who has finally got pregnant after fertility treatment, there is also affirmation that losing a baby after a long struggle to conceive can feel like a compounded loss. By sharing these stories, Sheila's book fosters an understanding for the intense feelings of grief as well, quite simply, what you should do on a practical level if you experience a loss.

Hopefully it is consoling to know that there are certain feelings and issues that come up repeatedly. They are real, and normal, and it is only by talking about them more that we will progress knowledge and care.

They include:

- The challenge of the 'three-month rule' (i.e. the accepted practice of not telling people you're pregnant until the end of the first trimester). If you lose your baby early, it can be very difficult for people to empathise because they didn't know you had anything to lose.

- The lack of language to describe this loss which can lead to an under-estimation of the feelings of grief it causes, as well as insensitive comments from people who do not understand it.

- All the unanswered questions – from did I do anything to make this happen; to would my baby have looked like me?

- The huge difficulty in being able to celebrate and enjoy a future pregnancy because of the fear that you might lose your baby again.

And the fact that men experience pregnancy loss too – their feelings and reactions may differ from women but they also suffer. It's great to see some honest and heartfelt contributions from men in this book. We definitely need more of that.

One thing is clear though and it echoes throughout – sharing your experience with others helps immensely. And although the pain may never go away - because the loss is real - it does lessen over time, especially if you allow yourself to experience the grief in whatever way you feel it, and get the support you need. However, it is also really important to recognise that there is no right or wrong way to experience grief; and that different people need different types of support. Whatever you feel and need is ok.

For me, the most significant thing about this book is that if you are someone who has experienced pregnancy loss and baby loss, you will know that you are not alone as you read the stories collected here. And if you are someone who hasn't, you will hopefully understand it better, which will make you more able to support those going through it.

This is pregnancy and baby loss – it's hard and it hurts but it is also a part of human life. By acknowledging this, we make the world a more loving, life-affirming place.

Jessica Hepburn

Author of The Pursuit of Motherhood and 21 Miles;

Founder of Fertility Fest

www.jessicahepburn.com

Acknowledgements

This book and the 'This is' series it's part of, wouldn't exist if it wasn't for the women and men who are part of the most amazing and supportive community that ever existed. It wasn't until I joined Instagram after publishing: My Fertility Book – All the Fertility and Infertility Explanations you will ever need, from A to Z, that I realised what 'community' actually means. Although my journey to motherhood included three unsuccessful fertility treatment cycles, and an early pregnancy loss before it ended happily several years ago, it has helped me to accept the emotions that come with loss and are still part of me.

My thanks, firstly, go to my miracle, rainbow daughter Jessica, (a rainbow baby is one who's born after a loss). She means the world to me and is my reason for writing in order to help and support the trying to conceive and baby loss community. Secondly, each contributor saw my vision for this series and has kindly shared their experience to support you. I appreciate each and every one of them, especially as I've never met most of them face-to-face, only on Instagram.

So, in alphabetical order: Alex @wheneverybodymatters, Alison Ingleby @footprintsonourhearts, Anna Rapp @ tomakeamommy, Anthony and Jalina King @thissideofif, Arden Cartrette @ardenmcartrette, Cat Strawbridge @tryingyears, Erin Bulcao @mybeautifulblunder, @fertili_arty, Frankie Brunker @ thesepreciouslittlepeople, Gabriel Soh @lovecommadad, Helena Tubridy @helenatubridy, Jackie Figueras @jackiefigueras, Jodi Sky Rogers @thefertilemoon, Justine Bold @justinebold, Karen Hanson @fertilitycircle, Karmann Wennerlind @ karmannwennerlind, Katie Ingram @withoutottilie, Dr Katy Huie Harrison PhD @khuieharrison, Katy Jenkins @ thejstartshere, Lauren Juggler Crook, Lauren @truths_of_ miscarriage, Lianne Baker, Lisa Sharrock @stillamama, Lucy @_mother_of_one_, Monica Bivas @monicabivas, Nicola Salmon @fatpositivefertility, Nora @thislimboland, Sharna Southan @sharnasouthan_coaching, Sophie Martin

11

@the.infertile.midwife, Suzanne Minnis @thebabygaim and Yuen Kwan Li @over40_tryingforababy.

If you would like to connect with any of these lovely people, there's a 'Resources' section at the back of this book.

The book cover has been illustrated by the author of IF: A Memoir of Infertility, Sheila Alexander, who was so supportive and patient as I stumbled to explain what I wanted for this book and the series. We both very much hope you relate to the couple on the front with their now grown up fur-baby. For more information visit her website: www.sheilaalexanderart.com or follow her on Instagram @sheilaalexanderart.

Like the other books in the series, I've included some illustrations in the hope that they bring some comfort to you if you're going through any loss. Illustrator and author, Phillip Reed, created the illustrations for *My Fertility Book* and for the other *This is* books. He can be contacted on philr@live.co.uk and Instagram @the_phillustrator.

I'd also like to thank the following people who have encouraged and supported me to put my *This Is* series of books together: my parents John and Freda, Paul Lamb, Judy Marell, Michelle Starkey, Claudia Sievers, Angie Conlon, Maria Bagao, Heidi Fitch, Melissa Werry, Sue Monaghan, Carla McMahon, contributors from the other books and my author writing group.

Contents

Contents

Introduction

I'm so sorry that you're reading this book because you've lost your baby during pregnancy. Please let me give you a virtual hug because few experiences can compare to the pain and trauma of the death of your precious baby. You may also be reading this because someone you care about has gifted the book to you, or maybe it was recommended so that you can understand why someone experiences grief at all stages of trying to have a baby.

Pregnancy loss happens after a natural conception and often a woman doesn't know she's had a pregnancy loss because her period is only a couple of days late. It can also occur after fertility treatment, such as IUI (intrauterine insemination) and IVF (in-vitro fertilisation). Stillbirth can also happen whether the baby was conceived naturally or through fertility treatment.

After our second ICSI (intracytoplasmic sperm injection – like IVF but a sperm is injected into the egg to fertilise it rather than letting the sperm do the fertilising), cycle for unexplained infertility, my husband and I got our first ever positive pregnancy test result. Within minutes I was already planning a future with our child. We had the much anticipated six-week scan where we would see our baby. Only we didn't. There wasn't a baby anymore. The grief, sadness, and shock were huge. One minute I was pregnant and within a blink of an eye, I wasn't.

There wasn't even time to say goodbye. I'd had no bleeding, no cramps so we were totally unprepared for this news. We hadn't told many people I was pregnant and it happened just before Christmas, so I found myself telling family and friends that I'd had a loss. Some were supportive but others didn't seem to acknowledge that we'd lost our precious baby. Maybe this was because they hadn't heard the good news first. We were very blessed that on our next ICSI (Intracytoplasmic Sperm Injection) cycle, our two-cell, two-day-old embryo became our rainbow baby, Jessica.

I found out several years later that although we went on to

have a baby, I'd suffered PTSD (post-traumatic stress disorder) after the pregnancy loss. A study by researchers at Imperial College London*, UK, found that four in ten women reported symptoms of PTSD three months after early pregnancy loss and ectopic pregnancy, (where the baby develops outside of the womb, often in a Fallopian tube).

If you've had a pregnancy loss or your baby has been stillborn, there are so many emotions you'll feel - numbness, shock, emptiness, anger, sadness, guilt, and many more. Grieving is important after any loss, and there's no right or wrong way to do this, nor is there a time limit. Everyone is different – some won't want to talk or see anyone, whereas others may find it helps to talk and be around people.

Experiencing loss in pregnancy is life-changing, and like a lot of people when this happens, I wanted to give something back to those who also found themselves on this path, to offer help and support.

As I'd also been through infertility, I wanted to support both communities, as they are often interlinked. Coming from a medical background – I was a nurse and midwife many years ago – I appreciated that understanding the medical terms whilst going through infertility is difficult, so I wrote my first book: My Fertility Book: all the fertility and infertility explanations you will ever need, from A to Z and published it in 2018. It's a jargon-free glossary of over two hundred medical and non-medical terms, with illustrations to help explain, accompanied by cartoons to bring a smile to your face.

Most fertility terms have acronyms or are abbreviated, such as AMH, BBT, and 6DP5DT, and are often used on social media, forums, online groups, and websites. So, I wrote a free eBook called: The Best Fertility Jargon Buster: the most concise A-Z list of fertility abbreviations and acronyms you will ever need and it can be download here: www.mfsbooks.co.uk

After finding the Instagram communities, I was so pleased to see how supportive and caring everyone was towards each other. Sadly, pregnancy loss and baby loss are still taboo subjects in most societies, so finding someone who has experience from your own social network isn't always easy. Even though my pregnancy loss was many years ago and I now have a daughter, I was comforted by what people were writing. And it was whilst reading these posts that gave me the idea of collating all these lovely, warm, supportive, virtual hugging words into a book.

All the contributors have experienced a loss, sometimes several losses, and they saw my vision for the book and the series – none of us wants anyone to feel alone at such a traumatic time in our lives. They share their emotions honestly, what helped or didn't help them, practical advice, and how they are also helping others in this community. Please note that some of what is contained within each individual contribution includes details of their loss and the aftermath that might prove upsetting or triggering, but they share these details and what they went through in the hope that those reading it might feel less alone if they have ever been through similar. You don't have to read the book from cover to cover, please do take a break and return to the book if it's proving emotionally taxing, and remember, some contributions will be more relevant or helpful to you than others.

I also hope the books help people outside of the baby loss community – family, friends, hospital staff, and other healthcare professionals – to better understand what people go through.

There are many different ways to find the support you need, such as counselling, online communities, organisations, podcasts, support groups, and books like this. Having all this support in a book means you don't have to search around on the internet - which will save you from seeing triggering adverts, such as maternity wear and baby equipment - you especially don't want to see these whilst going through this traumatic time.

With Love

Sheila xx

Visit my website at www.mfsbooks.com

*https://www.imperial.ac.uk/news/194715/miscarriage-ectopic-pregnancy-trigger-long-term-post-traumatic/

17

A letter to someone who has experienced a loss

Dear Friend

I'm so very sorry that you're reading this book because you've lost your baby. Regardless as to how many weeks pregnant you were, you already had hopes and dreams and planned a future with your baby. Everyone's experience is unique, but from seeing those two pink lines or the words 'You're 2-4 weeks pregnant', you've already connected with your son or daughter. Maybe you only saw them as a tiny blip on the ultrasound scan or heard their heartbeat. Maybe you've been pregnant for many weeks, saw your baby develop on ultrasound scans, and felt your baby move, but now your baby has gone and left you behind. We all feel your pain and want you to know that you're not alone.

You cannot prepare yourself for a loss like this. How it happens is different for everyone. But how it feels emotionally is very similar for many. Everyone who's contributed to this book has experienced losing their baby. Some have lost more than one child. They know what it's like to be excited about being pregnant and then, seconds later, to be told their baby has died. How do you deal with having your happiness snatched away so brutally?

The first thing they'll tell you is that it isn't your fault. It wasn't because of something you did or didn't do. It wasn't because you ran for the bus or you had that extra cup of coffee. You couldn't have done anything to stop it happening. During the first trimester, one of the main causes of pregnancy loss is that the baby wasn't developing normally due to chromosomal abnormalities. Chromosomes come from the mother and the father, and abnormalities happen by chance. Late pregnancy losses can also be caused by chromosomal abnormalities, an underlying health condition you weren't aware of, or because you caught an infection. You may think your pregnancy loss was down to something you ate, drank, or did, such as sitting in a sauna or having sex, but it was likely coincidental. You certainly didn't cause your pregnancy loss by tempting fate, such as buying baby clothes, telling people, or because you were stressed. There's no link between stress, pregnancy loss and baby loss.

You're not alone as pregnancy loss and stillbirth are sadly quite common. One in four pregnancies ends in pregnancy loss, and the chance of a second pregnancy loss is fourteen to twenty-one percent. In the UK, stillbirth occurs in around one in two-hundred births, and in the US, it's roughly one in one-hundred-and-sixty births. You probably thought it was only you going through this because rarely do mothers or fathers tell others that they've experienced pregnancy loss, or that their baby died. Once you start to confide, you'll be surprised by how many people tell you that they've also had a pregnancy loss or they know someone who has. Both pregnancy and baby loss are still a taboo subject around the world, but this isn't right, and many organisations are trying to change this. There's also a huge baby loss community online, especially on Instagram, but many aren't aware of this until they look for some kind of support. It's often a huge but lovely surprise to find people talking about their pregnancy loss or baby loss.

We're all different, of course, and some people will want to talk a lot about their experiences, and others won't want to share. There's no right or wrong way, just do what feels best for you. And if initially, you don't want to tell anyone, but then a few weeks later you do, that's also fine.

Most people don't share that they're pregnant until they're at least twelve weeks gone, because society thinks that after twelve weeks, you're in the 'safe zone,' i.e. nothing will go wrong with your pregnancy. But we know there's no safe zone. For you, that cluster of cells was your dream, your future, you were already in love. The people you tell may struggle to understand why you're sad and why you think you've lost a baby, and this is often because they've had no relationship with your baby. They also haven't experienced the excitement of finding out that you're pregnant; instead, you're telling them about something that will never happen. They don't mean to be unsupportive, but it can be hurtful for you if they dismiss your grief and sadness, and say something insensitive like: "Isn't it good that you weren't more pregnant?" – No! You were pregnant with your baby. Full stop. Or "You can have another one." Maybe you can, but you wanted this baby.

Most importantly, we understand, and that's why we're sharing our personal experiences here in this book. We don't want you to think that you shouldn't feel grief, that you shouldn't talk about your baby who you didn't take home, that you shouldn't include them in your family. You, and your partner and any of your baby's siblings, are far more important at this time than anyone else, and if others don't understand, pop this book in their hands, make them a cuppa and give them a little time to read about other people's experiences. If they read about similar traumatic experiences to what you've been through, it will help them to empathise with your loss and break the silence around pregnancy and baby loss.

There are many ways to find the support that's right for you and with every contribution is the person's name and/or Instagram link. If the contributor is also professionally helping the loss community, at the back of the book is a 'Resources' section in case you'd like to connect with them.

The most important thing to remember is that #youarenotalone – we are all here for you.

Much love

Sheila and the baby loss community xx

A letter to someone who hasn't experienced pregnancy or baby loss

Dear Friend

Thank you so much for opening this book. I, and the baby loss community, appreciate you taking the time to learn more about what it's like for someone to lose their baby, regardless of how old their baby was. It may surprise you to know that an estimated one in four pregnancies ends in pregnancy loss. Sadly, one in one hundred women in the UK has recurrent pregnancy loss, which means they'll potentially have three or more. Indeed, many women don't know that they've had a loss, only that their period was a couple of days late, but they hadn't taken a pregnancy test, so they don't know for certain. For women who have undergone fertility treatment, such as IVF (in-vitro fertilisation), they know when the embryo (a fertilised egg) was returned to their womb and they'll take a pregnancy test roughly two weeks later, if not before. Stillbirth in the UK occurs in around one in two-hundred births and in the US, roughly one in one-hundred-and-sixty births.

In this book, everyone has shared their emotions of loss, and some have also written about what they went through physically because they want to support others who are going through the same experience so they don't suffer alone, and also, so you aren't afraid to talk with them about their baby-loss and their son or daughter.

There are many 'losses' when it's a struggle to get pregnant and bring your baby home:

- A positive home pregnancy test that was short-lived and became a chemical pregnancy, blighted ovum, missed pregnancy loss, ectopic pregnancy, or early pregnancy loss – the woman or couple experienced the excitement of seeing a positive result only to have it snatched away.

- Molar pregnancy is when there's a chromosomal abnormality that occurs at the time of fertilisation – it's usually discovered during the twelve-week ultrasound scan when the heartbeat can't be seen and the placenta is abnormal. There's a risk the woman will develop choriocarcinoma and require chemotherapy, so she experiences grief at the loss of the baby and relief that the molar pregnancy was detected.

- Termination for medical reasons (TFMR), compassionate induction or medically based termination is when a much-wanted baby has a fatal or life-limiting condition, and the parent(s) decide to end the pregnancy – this is a tremendously difficult decision for parents to make and they experience significant grief and sadness.

- A late pregnancy loss happens between fourteen and twenty-four weeks of pregnancy – the parent(s) have seen their baby developing on their scans, have a scan or 3D photo, and have shared the exciting news with family and friends, so the loss is experienced by everyone.

- Stillbirth is when the baby dies in the womb before birth – in the UK after twenty-four weeks and in the US after twenty weeks of pregnancy. The loss of a baby this late into the pregnancy brings unimaginable pain – the mother will either have to give birth or have a caesarean when the baby is already fully-formed.

At four weeks pregnant when most women/couples see a positive pregnancy test, cells are creating the baby's brain. At six weeks the baby's heartbeat can be seen and heard on a vaginal ultrasound scan. At seven weeks, they can make jerky movements, and by twelve weeks you can tell if they're a boy or a girl.

I'm sure you can see now that any pregnancy loss, regardless as to how many weeks pregnant the woman was, means that the parent(s)-to-be think of their developing embryo as their baby, and will mourn and experience grief as if they'd already held their son or daughter in their arms. The most supportive thing you can do is acknowledge that and not dismiss their loss by perhaps saying, "You can have another" - it's crucial you remember that this couple wanted this baby; or "It was meant to be" – no parent should ever hear someone say these words to them.

You may not know the best way to support a family that has lost a baby and why should you if you haven't experienced a loss like this. Most of us didn't know what it was like until it happened to us. Please don't pretend nothing has happened; this is the worst thing you can do. Be guided by us; sometimes we'll retreat into ourselves, and might not want to attend gatherings. Don't be offended, it's nothing you've done, it's just the best thing for us at that time. We need to take care of our mental health. Remember too, that it wasn't just the mum who was pregnant, their partner will also be experiencing grief and sadness.

A man often deals with grief differently, but it doesn't mean he isn't as devastated. Don't forget that siblings, or other family members of the baby, will also be affected that their baby brother, sister or cousin has died, especially if they'd seen scan photos and talked to 'the bump'. If the parents or siblings want to talk, the best thing you can do is listen; don't try and fix it, don't tell them you know someone who went on to have a healthy baby after loss. And if they'd named their baby, talk about them by their name ... trust me, it won't make the parents feel any sadder than they already are. In fact, many say they love to hear people use their baby's name.

Although we're all on different journeys to have our longed-for babies, how we feel emotionally is often very similar. Hopefully, the contributions you'll read in this book will reveal this and either help you support the much-loved friend or relative who's going through this loss, or enable us to support you if you've been affected.

Much love,

Sheila and the baby loss community xx

Ten things you should never hear someone say

"It wasn't a proper baby"

"You'll be fine"

"You'll get over it"

"It's nature's way"

"It wasn't your time"

"Something must have been wrong and it's probably for the best"

"At least you can get pregnant, so you can have another baby"

"Don't worry, you can try again"

"Everything happens for a reason"

"Was it your fault?"

Sheila Lamb @fertilitybooks

Ten things you should hear someone say

"It wasn't your fault"

"I'm sorry for your loss"

"If you would like to talk about it, I'm here"

"Be gentle with yourself"

"This is sh*t and it will be sh*t for a while, but I promise you it will get better"

"It's OK to be sad and cry"

"I know it was early but it was still your baby"

"Your baby was loved"

"It's OK to be angry for as long as you want"

"Your baby will always be with you in your heart"

Sheila Lamb @fertilitybooks

Imagine if...

You'd never hear or see this baby's heartbeat at the ultrasound scan

You'd never make a pregnancy announcement on social media for this baby

You'd never felt this baby move in your womb

You'd never place your partner's hand on your growing belly so they could feel this baby move

You'd never attend this baby's baby shower

You'd never hear the midwife or doctor say "It's a girl" or "It's a boy"

You'd never tell this baby how much you love them

You'd never make a birth announcement on social media for this baby

You'd never hear this baby's first cry

You'd never give this baby their first cuddle

You'd never feel this baby's soft, warm skin against your skin

You'd never kiss this baby goodnight

You'd never feel this baby's hand hold onto your finger

You'd never see this baby's first smile or hear them coo

You'd never bought this baby their first Easter/Halloween/Christmas outfit

You'd never hear this baby say their first word

You'd never see this baby crawl for the first time

You'd never play tickle monster with this baby

You'd never see this baby reach out their arms to you for a cuddle

You'd never see this baby take their first steps

You'd never push this baby on the swing

You'd never buy this child their first pair of shoes

You'd never hear this child say "I love you mummy" or "I love you daddy"

You'd never cry when you take this child to their first day at nursery or first day at school

You'd never jump in muddy puddles with this child

You'd never see this child perform in their first nativity play

You'd never build a sandcastle or a snowman with this child

You'd never hear this child tell you what they want to be when they grow up

You'd never celebrate this child's exam results with them

You never look up to this child because they've grown taller than you

You'd never meet this child's first girlfriend/boyfriend

You'd never help this child arrange their marriage

Imagine if you didn't have all your memories of these precious moments with your child.

Imagine what it's like for me to know I'll never have these memories with this child.

Sheila Lamb @fertilitybooks

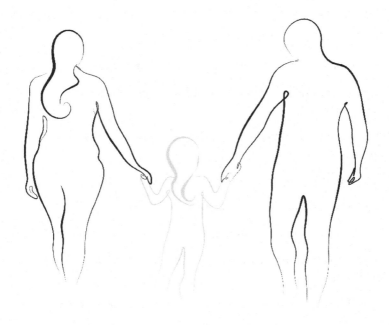

Losing a baby doesn't mean they are forgotten in the future

PREGNANCY LOSS

You lose your hopes and dreams

I never imagined trying to have a baby could be so difficult, so heart-breaking, so all-consuming, and some of the darkest moments of my life. I could never have imagined that I would lose three of our four babies – lose doesn't even seem to be the right choice of word, does it? It implies I carelessly left them somewhere. How could I be so reckless? I often wonder what could have been, what would our children have been like, would they be like their sister or completely different, would I have been a mother of three by now?

I've spent five of the past six years trying to have a family. I lost our first baby seven weeks into our pregnancy. It was such a shock; I'll never forget how frightened I felt and how much it hurt physically and emotionally. It was also incredibly isolating. I didn't know how long it would take to feel "normal" again, if it was usual to feel such intense grief, and how long I should take off work?

As I was packed off from hospital, incredibly traumatised with a packet of pain relief meds there was no mention of the mental toll losing our baby would take, and no suggestions of where to find support. No one followed up or checked on how I was getting on. It was "just one of those things" and "at least I knew I could get pregnant" – and that was that. I remember feeling that my baby wasn't just "one of those things," they were my everything. Three years later, we finally welcomed our daughter into the world after undergoing IVF for unexplained secondary infertility. Pregnancy after loss is frightening. You never fully allow yourself to believe this could be the time – it was only after my daughter arrived that I felt I could breathe again and accept she was "real".

I remember the midwife saying in the delivery suite shortly after her arrival, "You'll be ok next time, your body knows what it's doing now." I didn't believe her, but somehow a month before our daughter turned one, I found myself staring in disbelief at the positive pregnancy test in my hands.

At seven weeks, I went to the toilet and was greeted by the sight of blood. I lost our baby at home twelve hours later and I was completely shocked that this had happened again. As the midwife said, I thought my body now knew what to do. Again, I was told it was "just one of those things."

We had a family party that day and I went because I didn't want to be left alone at home. I was asked countless times by well-meaning relatives, "Isn't it about time you had another?" Each time I wanted to scream, "I've just lost our baby, please don't ask me," but instead, I smiled and nodded.

We decided to try again, and amazingly just two months later, I found myself pregnant once more. I was frightened beyond belief. Each hour felt like an eternity, just trying to get to the end of the day with our baby still alive. We made it to seven weeks – there was a strong heart beating away on our scan. Maybe this would be our time. We went for a follow-up scan at ten weeks, I'd had no bleeding, I felt so sick and exhausted and my tummy was already swollen. Within moments I could tell something was wrong. There was no heartbeat, our baby had died a week after our seven-week scan. I was devastated. A "missed" pregnancy loss seemed the hardest blow by far. How was I going to bounce back from this?

Baby loss can be incredibly isolating. For a long time, I felt so alone in my feelings. Should I feel such grief for these teeny-tiny lives? I was early into my pregnancies – but it's the hopes and dreams that you grieve for too – the vision of a future family life that's then so heartbreakingly torn away in an instant.

I felt ashamed of my body. Why couldn't it hold on to our precious and much-wanted babies? Why couldn't I do what others seemingly did so easily? I blamed myself; why couldn't I keep our babies safe? What was I doing wrong? I know now I wasn't to blame and sometimes there are no reasons, but it took a long time to reach that point of acceptance.

I'm learning to accept that sometimes there are no answers or reasons no matter how much we need them. I've also learnt that there's an inspiration in meeting others who have been through similar experiences.

Even in the darkest moments of despair, good things can come. They may not arrive in the way you imagined, but you will find happiness once more.

Lucy @_mother_of_one_

When you lose a twin

The tumultuous emotions on discovering you're going to lose one of your twins during pregnancy can be incredibly difficult to comprehend. This is the story of my third pregnancy loss, during a pregnancy that did finally give us 'our little survivor' as we nicknamed her, after losing her identical twin at ten weeks.

All my pregnancy losses have followed rounds of IVF. The first two pregnancies were singletons. An early scan at eight weeks showed the first to be a missed pregnancy loss, the second we anticipated losing from the get-go due to low beta numbers on test day.

The circumstances surrounding pregnancy, and at the same time baby loss, (there must be a name for this), may be different for all, however, the result is the same – a little human whom we may already have created a lifetime of memories for is no longer there. No matter what stage or how the loss occurred they'll always be with you. You are their mother or father, grandparent or auntie still, and the impact of that should never be ignored.

When you lose a twin there can be additional feelings attached to the loss. What would happen to the dead baby inside me? Would it come out when I gave birth? I worried that my little survivor would be lonely in the womb and when she finally arrived into the world. Would the joy of looking at our healthy baby bring with it a constant reminder of what we'd lost. Would we always see the empty space beside her on her birthday, her first day at school and her graduation pictures, and all the other occasions that happen throughout a lifetime?

During our pregnancy, I shared our loss on social media and I was contacted by someone who was also that little survivor for her parents. She put my mind at rest, telling me she'd never felt lonely or felt any impact around not having her twin. Her reaching out was a gift to me at that time, and I hope if you've experienced this, hearing that will bring you some peace too.

As for feeling the loss day to day, I still do, sometimes. It doesn't take a special occasion for the grief to creep up on me, but equally, it doesn't cast a shadow over them either. We didn't officially name her lost sister, but sometimes I say the name I think she might have had alongside my daughter's and I miss her. I wonder what she would have looked like, and who she would have become. I feel sad that Wren doesn't have a little sibling here, especially as we may not be able to have another little brother or sister for her. I feel sad that we could have moved on from 'trying' for more if we'd had a readymade family of four.

With any loss, it's so important to get support. Research shows there's a deep-rooted connection between pregnancy/baby loss and mental health issues. Your recovery – because you will recover – will be helped enormously by realising this.

Following my first and second pregnancy loss, I sought counselling from a charity based in my hospital. I'll admit I didn't go immediately – not because I couldn't handle it myself, rather that I didn't realise what an impact the loss had on me until I started to unravel. Once I did, I was so grateful for the time and support I received from the counsellor. I think the work I'd done previously helped when we had our third pregnancy loss. That and the huge trying to conceive and baby loss community I'm lucky to have found on Instagram.

Whoever you talk to – whether it be to friends, family, internet 'strangers', or a professional – make sure you talk. There are others out there going through similar experiences and sometimes that can be the most powerful thing to hear – "me too, you are not alone."

Cat Strawbridge @tryingyears

I don't mind the scars that have been left behind

When you've watched your precious embryo being carefully placed into your uterus during an IVF (in-vitro fertilization) transfer, the last thing you expect to happen is an ectopic pregnancy. Yet here I was four weeks later in the hospital waiting room, working my way through a pile of magazines with a pain in my side and my left shoulder becoming increasingly worse.

I'd been waiting for blood test results for most of the day, leaving hospital only briefly to get a bite to eat at midday – a cheese scone, half of which I'd accidentally dropped on the floor. By the time my name was called, I was doubled over in pain and could barely hobble.

At 4 p.m. I was finally given a scan; the pregnancy was indeed ectopic and my fallopian tube had ruptured so I needed urgent surgery. I remember apologising, "I hope my surgery won't delay anybody else," And then I burst into tears as the doctor showed me the scanned image on the screen. I composed myself quickly as suddenly the room became a flurry of activity.

I must have seen at least ten different members of staff in the space of half an hour. I was quickly briefed about the surgery and its risks: "Ectopic pregnancies can be fatal – don't worry, you should be fine." I was weighed, measured, helped into a gown and surgical socks, and bundled into a hospital bed.

"What time did you last eat?"

"12 pm, I dropped half my scone…"

"Do you have any allergies?" "Who is your next of kin?" "I'm just putting a cannula into your arm." "I'm sorry to ask but what would you like to happen to the remains? Please sign here to confirm." "What time did you last eat?"

"12 pm, I dropped half my…"

"I'm just going to put this gel on, it might feel cold." "Please sign to consent here." "How many weeks pregnant are you?"

"What time did you last eat?"

"12 pm, I dropped half my scone."

At 4:30 p.m I was wheeled down to theatre. "Is this your first pregnancy?"

"It's an IVF baby."

Sympathetic murmurs. It was cold in the theatre. I was only really thinking of myself at this point. More tears. Two smiling female nurses squeeze a hand each and say things which sound reassuring. The kindly anaesthetist used gentle humour to put me at ease, and a couple of hours later it was over. The surgery went well and I will be forever grateful to the NHS (National Health Service) for their love and care.

In the weeks and months that followed, I felt the heartbreak, frustration and deep sense of grief that can stem from all forms of pregnancy loss. The physical recovery took time (drinking peppermint tea works wonders with the gas pain), and the shock from the trauma of it all also lingered as I would spontaneously cry most days.

Talking to other women with similar stories through our Instagram page has been invaluable. As with all life experiences, it's such a comfort to know we're not alone. I don't mind the scars that have been left behind. They are a reminder of how hard we've tried to grow our family.

@fertili_arty

Pregnancy loss tore our friendship apart

"You're going to miscarry." Those were the exact words out of my friends' mouth. Not just any friend either, my best friend of seventeen years. We met at uni. She thought I was a nerd and I thought she was a snob, and yet we formed an incredibly close bond, telling each other everything. We studied, travelled and hung out together. Even when I moved from Sydney to London and back, and she moved to New York, we always stayed in touch. And each time we face-timed it was like we'd just spoken only yesterday, even though months might have passed.

She never wanted children, she always stated that she didn't have any maternal instincts. She told me that from day one and that never changed, even after she got married to someone who desperately wanted children. So, you can imagine my utter shock when she insisted on calling me while I was on holiday in Croatia with my husband to tell me she was pregnant. Fifteen weeks pregnant! Not only did she keep this a secret, but she'd told everyone including her HR team at work before me. Her maternity leave was approved before I even had a clue.

I was so hurt because only six months earlier, I'd told her I was pregnant. Only I'd told her at six and a half weeks once we'd been to our first ultrasound to confirm it all. The first thing she said to me was, "You're going to miscarry, lots of people lose their first." Devastatingly, two weeks later I did. I was so upset that a friend who never wanted a baby was now having a baby, and she waited so long to tell me when we'd shared every single thing for nearly two decades. I felt betrayed.

Our friendship changed forever that day and never recovered. She cut me out of her entire pregnancy, and to this day I still don't know why, although I suspect my pregnancy loss had everything to do with it. It divided us, sent us down different paths in life.

I asked her for ultrasound pictures and bump-date pictures and she always promised to send them but she never did. She suddenly became too busy to chat and I stopped receiving messages between calls. She didn't even tell me when her little one was born. I have no idea whether she had a boy or girl, what their name is or what they looked like.

Through pregnancy loss I lost my best friend. However, I also gained something so incredibly valuable – an amazing TTC (trying to conceive) community. We share deeply and openly, supporting one another. We commiserate with and celebrate each other. It's a club that I never in my wildest dreams thought that I'd be a member of, but now, I'm so glad I am. They just get it! We just get it.

So please don't ever feel that you're alone or have to suffer in silence. You're not and you don't. We've got you.

Nora @thislimboland

Second trimester loss

Firstly, I'm so sorry that you need to read this book. Baby loss is completely devastating and I wouldn't wish it on my worst enemy. Please seek professional help if you need it as there are some great resources out there, including Sands (Stillbirth and Neonatal Death charity).

I'm not an expert in baby loss, however, I have both cared for families during their darkest hour, and also said goodbye to two of my own precious babies. The following is a collection of thoughts that I have gathered along the way.

I would like to wish you my heartfelt congratulations. Congratulations are often absent after the death of a baby. But you created the most beautiful precious being, who has only ever known love, and that is deserving of praise.

There will always be the time before, and the time after, and losing something so priceless alters your life in ways that are beyond imagining. I used to hate phrases like 'time is a great healer' or 'it gets easier with time'. The loss still hurts just as much as it did on that very first day. However, you'll get better at dealing with the emotions.

Be gentle and respectful towards your partner. They're grieving too and their grief may look very different to yours. You're joined together as the parents of your child and you'll both continue to parent your baby even after their death.

Feel free to remember your baby however you see fit, whether that's lighting a candle on their birthday or talking about them every day. There's no right or wrong way to honour your child.

I don't wish the memory of my sons to be one of sadness or devastation, and therefore I think of the gifts that my sons have given me. They've bestowed upon me the gift of motherhood, the gift of empathy and the gift of unconditional love, for which I'm eternally grateful.

One of the most challenging things to navigate post-loss is the,

"Do you have any children?" question. You don't owe the asker any details of your life that you aren't ready to share. You're not denying your child's existence just because you don't share them with a stranger. And on the other hand, you have a right to be proud of your child, the same way that parents with living children are.

All of your feelings are valid. Even the 'ugly' ones. It's perfectly reasonable to be resentful, angry, jealous and sad. It's also normal to feel numb. I felt like a plug had been pulled out and there was a deep well of emotions, and that my feelings ran a lot deeper and more intensely then they'd been previously.

Sadly, some of the people you thought were friends will disappear after the death of your baby. This is not a reflection on you, so instead hold tight to the friends and family that do step up.

Finally, please note that it is possible to feel happiness again after the loss of your baby; that you will smile again, and the sun will shine on your life once more.

Grief is temporary, but love is forever.

Sophie Martin @the.infertile.midwife

I didn't do anything wrong

When I found out I was pregnant for the first time I was in utter shock. After trying to conceive for three years and having gone through three failed IVF cycles, I was finally pregnant, and it happened naturally. My husband and I were elated.

About a week after finding out, I started to spot blood and panic set in immediately. I rang the Early Pregnancy Clinic and booked in for an early scan. We hoped it was just implantation bleeding but the anxiety never left me during those first few days. Then the day before my scan, I bled heavily. I was so scared that we went straight to A&E. I sat in reception and couldn't stop crying; the worry was overwhelming. I had a scan but the Doctor said I was around five weeks rather than seven. I felt like we were left in limbo; it might be bad news or it might be fine. We had to return in a week to find out.

Those seven days were the worst of my life, waiting to find out if our baby was still alive. I had no more bleeding, so I took that as a good sign. But I was still terrified sitting in the waiting room of the Early Pregnancy Clinic. I didn't want to look at the posters on the wall that said 'one in four pregnancies end in a pregnancy loss,' but I couldn't stop myself. I hoped more than anything that it wouldn't be us, but when we were called in, it wasn't good news. The midwife was so lovely and I'll never forget her kindness towards us when she said, "I'm so sorry, but there's no baby there anymore, just an empty sac and lots of blood in your womb." The sac was empty and so was my heart. I'll never forget that feeling of profound loss. I already loved my baby and I didn't get to say goodbye. I never got to hold my child and tell them they meant the world to me. She explained that I'd bleed heavily over the next few days. That thought was horrible. My husband grabbed my hand tightly as we walked out of the room. He anticipated my oncoming breakdown of tears and supported me walking down the corridor. We drove to a little spot we love and sat in the car talking and crying.

After four days nothing had happened. I didn't have any more bleeding which I was expecting and I couldn't take it anymore, so I rang the hospital to ask if I could be booked in for a D&C. I couldn't stand the thought that my baby had gone and I was carrying around what was left inside me. I went to hospital a few days later and had the operation. It was such a sad time as it seemed so final. It was goodbye. Afterwards, I felt it was time to grieve and strongly felt that I needed to mark the loss of our baby. So, I wrote a letter to my unborn child and kept it in a special box that I still have. I went through turbulent emotions at the time such as guilt, sorrow and loneliness.

My husband was also devastated but he often didn't show how he really felt. I was frustrated because I didn't see in him the despair and sadness I was experiencing, but I know now it was there, just hidden inside. One day I found him upset and it broke my heart in two. I appreciated more than ever how strong he'd always been for both of us. He's my rock. It's so important to remember that losing a baby is devastating for men as well.

At the time I felt like a failure. It's taken me a long time to realise that it wasn't my fault and that I couldn't have done anything differently. Support from loved ones is so important, and I'll always be grateful for the wonderful friends and family I have. Each hug, chat, letter or text built me up again, so I could absorb all that love and good energy. It reminded me that I wasn't alone.

Unfortunately, pregnancy loss does happen to a lot of women but that doesn't make it any easier when it happens to you, and it doesn't make your loss any less devastating. We went on to have a beautiful daughter two years later, but I'll never stop thinking about the baby we lost. Our first pregnancy and first baby will always be in our hearts.

Suzanne Minnis @thebabygaim

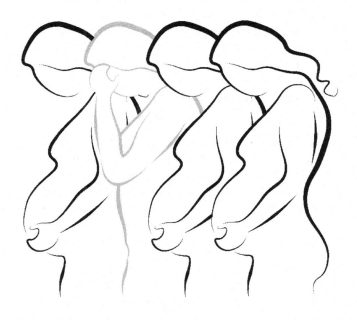

1 in 4 pregnancies results in pregnancy loss

Discuss your feelings openly and honestly

There's no such thing as being 'a bit pregnant.' When you get a positive pregnancy test, you're fully pregnant, and losing your baby at any stage during those nine months is devastating. Everyone experiences loss and grief differently – even in a relationship, partners react differently at various stages. Some need time to grieve and others are ready to try and conceive again. There are no hard and fast rules, which makes pregnancy loss even harder to navigate because how can you ever be prepared?

On the outside, you may appear fine, glad of the normalcy of being back at work. Your body may still feel pregnant and there are markers people may skirt around – maternity leave and due dates. Healing needs to happen on both physical and emotional levels, however long or quickly that happens.

My clients find it helps to understand why they feel whatever it is they're feeling at a particular time. This doesn't change those feelings, but it prepares them to feel safer and more comfortable in triggering situations.

People want to help but quite often manage to say unhelpful things. Even when their intentions are good, these comments can trigger overwhelming emotions, just when your resilience is at its lowest ebb. Knowing how to self-regulate emotions after the trauma of pregnancy loss can give you back a sense of control.

Find someone to talk to who hears and validates your experience without trying to 'fix the problem', nor launches into their own narrative. Family and friends may be all you need as they understand what you're going through. A professional counsellor or EMDR, (Eye Movement Desensitisation and Reprocessing) therapist can support you, believe in you, and hold a safe space, validate your feelings and walk you through a trusted process. Believe me, it's an honour to be there with you. You learn to treat yourself more compassionately at a time when sadness and fear can erode self-confidence. Hypnotherapy and EMDR give you the tools to reduce overwhelming feelings, while feeling safe inside the storm of challenging emotions. These aid a natural process and don't mean you're forgetting or obliterating this pregnancy loss. You're learning to live with it as part of your family narrative, honouring this little one, and preparing for another pregnancy if you want it and when you feel ready.

A client told me it was six months after her pregnancy loss that she asked her husband how he felt about their loss. Men may sometimes feel side-lined after a pregnancy loss and benefit from a listening ear outside the family/friend circle.

Shame and guilt about the 'loss' come up time and time again for my clients – as though somehow, they could have done something differently to preserve their pregnancy. You're a warm vibrant human being and you're allowed to have feelings. Give yourself full permission to have them all! Pushing away emotions or burying them down deep inside only stores them up for later.

Fear of conceiving after pregnancy loss is natural. Why wouldn't you worry about it? Discussing your myriad feelings honestly takes a weight off, and lets you re-centre yourself more easily.

Helena Tubridy @helenatubridy Esme's story

After pregnancy loss; some things I wish I'd known

Includes an excerpt from the blog: 'How to Deal with Miscarriage: seven things I wish I'd known'

Figuring out how to deal with pregnancy loss, both during and after the horrifying experience, IS REALLY HARD. One in four pregnancies ends in loss – and yet, because pregnancy loss has been a relatively taboo subject for so long, we've only recently begun to have conversations about it. After pregnancy loss, what to do next becomes even more confusing.

There are many things I wish I'd known that could have saved me so much heartache post-loss. For example, I wish someone had given me a script* for how to say "no" to a baby shower. I wish someone had talked to me about the struggle of coping with loss, and about how healing a pregnancy loss memorial can be. I wish someone had told the people around me how to help. If only they'd known what not to say. A rule book would've helped them.

No one tells you about the practical things you need to do after pregnancy loss, so that your heart isn't broken day after day. The following are four of the seven tips from my blog that I wish someone had given me.

1. Clear your Internet browser cache and cookies

You probably know that your data is being logged. Any website you browse, Google is collecting data, learning what you're interested in and providing the website owner with information about you. Is this creepy? Yes. Is it the world we live in? Also, yes. That's why when you search for something or click on a Facebook ad, suddenly you see that very thing EVERYWHERE. Because marketing is targeted towards you.

After a pregnancy loss or stillbirth, this is a super tricky issue to navigate. Why? Well, you've likely been looking up things that are related to babies. Even if you've searched for things like: 'pregnancy symptoms', 'morning sickness' or 'due date calculator,' you're going to start seeing ads for baby items on websites you visit. And let's be honest, you probably don't want to see this. I know I didn't. By clearing your browser cache and cookies, you can avoid getting these unwanted ads popping up on any website you're looking at. Remember, all your devices talk to each other, so you want to clear your browser cache, cookies and history on your phone, tablet and computer. No more ads for things you can't emotionally bear to see.

2. Update your loss on pregnancy apps

Did you put the date of your last missed period into The Bumps app as soon as you saw two lines? If you did this with any app - Glow, Ovia, What to expect, Pregnancy Tracker etc, then you're likely getting updates from them. And you're probably not too thrilled when you get a push notification on your phone telling you that your baby is the size of a pea. To save you this heartache, and the cost of replacing your phone after you smash it, these apps have mechanisms that allow you to 'Report a loss'; those were usually the words I saw, although it may vary between apps. Make sure you take the time to report your loss to every app you joined, otherwise the updates will continue.

3. Remove yourself from pregnancy groups

If an app is a good one, reporting a loss will also unsubscribe you from their mailing list. But unfortunately, this isn't always the case. To be on the safe side, give your partner or a friend you trust, temporary access to your email. Tell them what apps you were on and they can search for any emails from those apps, and unsubscribe you from their mailing lists. If you've joined any pregnancy Facebook groups or follow any pregnancy-related Instagram hashtags, leave them. You can always go back later, but I promise you, it's not worth the heartache now.

4. Put someone else in charge of the mail around your due date time

This is likely the most surprising item on this list. Buckle up and listen to this bullsh*t. Apparently, when you're pregnant, certain apps, website and even OB offices (or so I'm told) will share your data with different companies. You heard me. Nothing is safe. I gave up on privacy a long time ago, so I'm honestly fine with it, but it can manifest in ways you'd never imagine.

After my first loss, I'd done my best to figure out how to cope with this loss and I thought I'd covered all my bases. I unsubscribed from all the emails, left all the 'due in June' groups, and reported the losses to all my apps. When my due date rolled around, Husband and I left home because I wanted to be away. We went to Maine, and we had a ceremony to honor all the pregnancies we'd lost up to that point, (three at that time). It was both a fun and cathartic trip and was exactly what I needed.

Then we came home and found a box on our doorstep. It never occurred to me to ask Husband to get it. I grabbed the key, opened the door and nearly collapsed on the floor when I saw it. It was a cruelly heart-wrenching, 'Welcome baby' box from Similac, full of formula samples and coupons.

F*** you, Similac. Sorry, not sorry.

I have no idea how they got my information or my due date, but they did. Other women in my recurrent pregnancy loss group complain about this constantly as well. Until I figure out how to stop it and let you all know, I beg of you, I plead with you... leave every box at the door and every item in the mailbox when you're coming near to, and after, your due date. You'll receive coupons and congratulations and it will rip your heart to shreds.

I'm sorry and I hope someday it doesn't. But for now, please, I beg of you, don't check your own mail.

*Please email me if you would like this script.

Dr Katy Huie Harrison PhD @khuieharrison
(Link to the blog: https://undefiningmotherhood.com/how-to-deal-with-miscarriage/)

There's no right or wrong way to feel after pregnancy loss

There's nothing in this world that anyone can say to take away the pain of pregnancy loss. There are no magic words that make everything better. If there was, I would say them a thousand times over.

When I got pregnant, I was so excited. I thought 'I'm going to have a baby.' It never crossed my mind that something could go wrong until it did go wrong. I was blissfully unaware of possible complications and I didn't know just how common pregnancy loss is. I certainly know that hearing the phrase, "It's more common than you think," doesn't make anyone feel better, as every single loss experience is different. They say one in four pregnancies ends in pregnancy loss, but you're a person not a statistic.

When I first had my pregnancy loss, I shut down. I didn't want to talk or think about it. I just wanted to bury my head and hope it all went away. But that didn't work. I was drowning in sadness and found myself getting worse, not better. There's no right or wrong way to feel, and there were times I felt so lonely. So, I sought online help and discovered women just like me who want to feel heard. And I've never felt more supported than by the Instagram community.

There's no real way to 'get over' this loss. How can someone really ever get over the loss of the tiny life they love so much. Instead you have to try, as hard as it may be, but try to see a little good in every day. Accept that you're grieving and talk. Talk to anyone who will listen, talk to a friend, talk to family, talk to a woman online who's been through the same thing! Do not be ashamed of your story. Talking helped me feel less guilty, less at fault. Guilt will be an emotion you're likely to feel at some point. You'll ask yourself a lot of 'what ifs?' "What if I did something wrong?" But you're not to blame. In most cases, there's nothing anybody could have done to prevent your loss.

I've often found myself living in a future that no longer exists. Thinking what my baby would have looked like, and I found myself holding my belly thinking 'I should be thirty weeks now,' and 'my clothes shouldn't fit now.' This is a really hard mindset to get out of, and if I'm honest, I'm not quite there yet. But that's okay, healing is not linear. There's no set timeline to how long healing should take. It's ok if some days you have your life together and the next day you do nothing but cry. Allow yourself to cry, scream if you have to. These raw emotions show how much it meant to you and how much love you have to give, and hopefully, one day…

One quote that has always resonated with me is: 'I don't want to forget; I want to be okay with remembering.'

Remember your baby, remember the pain, but stay strong. You are stronger than you think.

Lauren @truths_of_miscarriage

Do you want to see my baby?

Based on an Instagram post from 10 October 2019

I want to share this info on my mental health during my journey. My tears well up thinking of this time in my life. It still feels real and like yesterday.

* This is a sensitive post. *

In August 2009, I sat in my bathroom looking at my miscarried baby yet again in my underwear. It was number eight – my fourth pregnancy loss this year. I scooped it up and placed it in a zip-lock bag. I must have held it for an hour crying, wondering if this was as far as I'd get with my pregnancies. Six weeks was my longest.

I thought back to earlier that day when someone asked me when I was going to have kids. I smiled brightly and said, "Hopefully someday!" Now, in my grief, I placed the bag in my purse and decided I was going to carry it around with me. I told myself that the next person who asked me that question, I was going to take my baby out and show them, saying: "I do have a baby. Do you want to see my baby? I can't seem to carry my baby to full term.? It's six weeks old. Don't you think my baby is beautiful?"

I carried that bag around for days. I looked at it a thousand times. I couldn't let it go. Luckily, no one asked me that question.

Thinking back to that time, I was at an all-time low. My losses had taken me to a whole other level of depression. Infertility can break you. I was broken. I'm thankful for a loving heavenly Father who was aware of me. We moved to Seattle four months later where I got help for my depression. It's also where I got my answers to why I kept losing my babies.

Four and a half years later and one more loss on from that scary time, I held my full-term baby boy in my arms.

This journey can break you, but don't let it keep you broken. I am proof you need to keep fighting even through the darkest times. Please, don't give up. I promise it's worth it. I'm here if you need me.

Karmann Wennerlind @karmannwennerlind

Pregnancy loss and fat people

Based on the blog: 'Pregnancy loss when you are fat'

Suffering from pregnancy loss when you are fat is not the same as someone in a smaller body.

For those of us in fat bodies, the message we're given is still very raw and very blunt; our bodies are the reason that we cannot maintain a healthy pregnancy, and if we could only lose weight, then we would be able to have a healthy pregnancy.

Even if no-one has said this to you before, I can guarantee the thought has crossed your mind, or you've been worried that others are thinking it. It's so normal for us to try and find a reason for this grief so we can make sense of it now, and avoid similar in the future.

But it's not your body's fault; you didn't lose this pregnancy because you are fat.

I know this may be hard to believe, especially as this is the story we are told. No matter the reason why it happened, you're worthy of appropriate and respectful care. You're a human being, and you deserve a level of healthcare that treats you like one.

There are no known ways of reducing further pregnancy losses specifically, but what you can do is look after yourself in the best way you can right now. This will be different for everyone but I always recommend that people:

- ensure they're getting enough rest

- ensure they're eating enough

- find a way to move their body in a way that feels good.

You don't have to throw yourself into a diet right now.

Supporting your mental health after a pregnancy loss

Acknowledge the grief

Experiencing any kind of pregnancy loss is a form of grief. No matter where you were in your pregnancy, not only did you lose your baby, but you lost your future with your baby. You lost the day you thought you'd bring your baby home, the time you thought you'd spend together in the baby's newly decorated nursery, every future memory you thought you'd make as a family. Even though you never met your baby, it's okay to grieve all that you lost.

Be OK feeling ALL THE EMOTIONS

Your emotions will fluctuate; they might change daily or even minute by minute. You might feel sad, angry, frustrated and hopeless all in one breath, and that's okay. You don't have to bottle anything up. It's important to express whatever emotions are there.

Honour your needs

In the same way that your emotions will change, your needs will change too. Sometimes you'll need physical closeness with your partner or a friend; sometimes you'll need to be alone; sometimes you'll need the release of sobbing your heart out, and sometimes that need will be a large glass of wine. Honour those needs. Trust that you'll know what you need at any moment and go with it. Ask yourself regularly: "What do I need now?" and ensure you're meeting those needs.

What story are you telling yourself?

When you've healed a little and are ready to explore, dig into the stories that you're telling yourself about your experience with pregnancy loss. What are you making this experience mean about you? Are you telling yourself that you'll never be able to have a healthy pregnancy? Do you believe that you caused your pregnancy loss? Do you believe that it's your body's fault? Are you afraid to get pregnant again because you believe you'll have another loss? Think about those stories that are based on facts and those that are created from things others have told you or that you've told yourself. Acknowledging those beliefs is the biggest step towards changing them. What do you want to believe instead?

The one thing I want you to take away from all of this is that you're worthy of becoming a parent and you're worthy of receiving the care that you need in order for this to happen.

Nicola Salmon @fatpositivefertility

(Link to the blog: http://nicolasalmon.co.uk/pregnancy-loss-when-you-are-fat/)

Men suffer to

Based on the blog: 'Father's Day on the rocks: a male perspective of infertility and miscarriage' from 'This Side of IF'

Father's Day 2015, I was told I was going to be a dad. I was excited.

As quickly as it came, it was gone. A week later, my wife and I were in the ER being treated for pregnancy loss. That's when I hit an emotional breaking point. I did what I could to comfort my wife, but I didn't know how to process my feelings or understand what I felt. We had been trying to conceive for over a year and late 2014, we'd had some infertility tests that showed I had poor sperm quality. However, this pregnancy we'd conceived naturally. I did little research as to what was going on as I figured my wife had done enough for both of us. I assumed it must be my fault; my low-quality sperm couldn't make a baby. I was mortified.

After the pregnancy loss I began to use alcohol to destress. Over the course of a month I rapidly deteriorated, my drinking got worse and in a fit of blind rage, I left my wife. She deserved better. I moved in with a friend who lived about ten miles away, and we drank and drank and drank. I tried to maintain a 'normal' life; I went to work and college, but both suffered because of my pain. I went from being a Dean's list student to barely scraping by with a 'D'. I showed up to work late most days, and usually left early. After about three weeks my boss fired me because I didn't show up for work. To my knowledge I wasn't supposed to be at work, but during this time I failed to check the schedule. I came and went as I pleased.

With some help from a tough love childhood pastor, I was able to recover and put my life back together. He was never afraid to seek out the broken, and his tall, burly stance was the opposite to his kind heart. He brought me back into the church, prayed over me and showed me that no matter how low I felt, God still loved and cared for me. He shared his own rough past with me. He started coaching me through the emotions I'd felt about the pregnancy loss, and helped me to process my actions. Even though I wasn't yet the Anthony I had previously been, I asked my wife for forgiveness, and a month after I'd left, she took me back and we are now happier than ever. I've learned to process my emotions positively using grounding and breathing techniques, as well as prayer and reading scripture. While pregnancy losses are still hard, I can tell you they're much harder when you're alone. Since our first loss we've suffered four more, and each time it tugs at my heart. But my wife is my rock and we both mutually support each other.

Infertility and loss have forever changed our marriage. While our relationship may never be the same as those first few years where having children wasn't constantly playing on our minds, we've never been stronger. We are more in tune with each other's emotions and needs. We mourn together, we hurt together, but no matter what, we are together.

Being a parent after infertility and a series of pregnancy losses gives me a different vision. Not everything is sunshine and rainbows. Everyone has struggles and more people than I ever realized share the same challenges we had. Fortunately, we now have three amazing little boys who were conceived naturally. They bring out the best in me and are my world. The pain and sorrow of those lost babies will always hold a sacred place in my heart. This Father's Day, I'm the proud dad of three sons and five angel babies.

Anthony King

(Link to the blog: https://thissideofif.com/male-perspective-infertility-miscarriage)

Commemorate your sweet little love

Hi Mama,

Yes, that's you, no matter the difference between the number of babies you've carried in your womb and how many you hold in your arms. For me, that difference is five pregnancy losses, all between four and eleven-weeks' gestation, and I want you to know something that took me years to learn and accept: your baby counts. Your baby is so loved and so are you.

I'm sorry for how alone you must feel in grieving the precious soul or souls you didn't get to meet. I'm sorry no one is sending you cards or bringing you home-made meals as you heal physically and emotionally from this simultaneous birth and death. I'm sorry for all the 'at least's,' 'the justs' and the 'maybe you shoulds' you've had to endure from the well-meaning but oh-so blissfully ignorant people in your life.

Here are a few ways to commemorate your sweet little love, counteracting those dismissive attitudes and showing the world that your baby forever has a place here, if only in your heart:

Name your baby. This has the power of transforming the grief of your loss into the joy of being your baby's mother. It moves your loss from a secretive place to one of connection and validation. Don't be afraid to choose a name you love or one you will her other people say. After such a devastating loss, it might surprise you how happy the sound of your babies name makes you feel. If you didn't get to learn their gender, you can choose a nickname or a gender-neutral name.

Choose a song, Bible verse, or quote to associate with your baby. Document why you chose them so you don't forget.

Hold a ceremony. This might be anything from a backyard memorial to a funeral depending on your grieving preferences and the gestation at which you lost your sweet babe. If you're having a ceremony at home, you might wish to include elements such as music, candles, scripture reading, a letter to your baby, or something physical to commemorate the ceremony, like pictures or a memory box. Our home cremation ceremony followed a reflective hike on a sunny spring day. It was my husband's idea to get out of the house instead of sitting around all day, waiting for the appointed ceremony time. I can honestly say the hike was peaceful and refreshing.

Plant a tree. This can be a beautiful reminder of your baby's life and a physical place to connect with him or her. If you have any remains or cremation ashes, you can use these when planting your tree. You might also wish to add a plaque, a bench, or chimes. If a tree is too permanent, a houseplant or a small flowering shrub are other options.

Choose a meaningful symbol. This could be stars, a certain type of flower, an animal, or even a color. Just like choosing a name, choosing a symbol to associate with your baby is a great way to continually feel his or her presence in everyday life. Keep the symbol to yourself as a special connection between you and your baby, or share it with others!

Purchase or create jewellery, art, or decorations. These are great ways to incorporate their name, birth date, due date, or any words or symbols you've chosen to associate with your baby. You could design a commemorative tattoo or make an ornament. Christmas can be an emotionally challenging time of year for those missing a loved one so making a Christmas ornament to uniquely represent your baby can be a therapeutic activity, and a way to include him or her in the holiday. There are also numerous options for memorial jewellery that can include cremation ashes, breastmilk, dehydrated placenta, or locks of hair.

If possible, involve your partner. Pregnancy loss can be detrimental to any relationship. By now, you may have learned the hard way that men and women grieve differently, and finding a way to grieve together might seem impossible. If it's possible to involve your partner, doing any of the above-listed activities together can be a sweet bonding experience and a reminder that he or she is hurting too, which can be oddly comforting in the sad world of pregnancy loss.

There are countless other ways to remember your baby from cuddling a teddy bear at night, (you wouldn't be the only one), to making a donation or starting a business in your baby's honor. You're a mama, and you bond with each of you babies is unique. Do what feels right for you, even if it might seem strange to others.

Jalina King @thissideofif

Pregnancy loss poems

Tomb

Foetus warm, wrapped inside,
I think of you with the longing of
'one day'.

Carrying you, for sixteen weeks
thinking you were safe.

Next time, over sooner.
Done by nine weeks.
No scan to etch in forever's mind,
all a pool of tears.

The one after, just fleeting moments,
— over within a week of starting.

They called it a chemical pregnancy.
One of the 'one in three'.

Two

The digital stick in my trembling hand confirms a dream. Two - three weeks pregnant. Only eight days after a blastocyst transfer, so it's strong. I am walking tall and very smiley, scared to believe it might be okay this time.

Activity becomes a distraction, planning and preparation. Need to know I've covered everything. Done all that might be possible. I could never forgive myself if I hadn't and something went wrong.

Blood tests every few days. Every precaution taken. Aspirin, heparin and lots of other medication. 40 mg prednisolone, plus drips every two weeks. Intralipids… soya and egg to confuse the errant natural killer cells and protect precious life.

Just before six weeks, blood clots the size of my palm. I think it's over, again. They scan. Two sacs; just one heartbeat. I think one is already gone.

Next scan

The next scan, two weeks later, so nervous, I don't want to look.

They tell us you are both still there. My heart skips a beat.

I smile; there are tears.

V/O A viable intrauterine DCDA twin pregnancy seen today.

Precious flutters of light as two heartbeats fight through bloody
clouds.

V/O Foetal heartbeat present – twin 1 and twin 2.

They give me a picture. Two little sacs resting against each other,
besides a long grey smudge.

V/O Between the two gestation sacs there is an echo poor
area seen which measures 17x25x12mm and is suggestive of a
haematoma.

The sonographer doesn't charge the normal fee.

Haematoma

One day my father cleans as my mother lies me down wiping away tears.

Bathroom floor flooded and mopped, again.

Each time, stuck … unable to read or concentrate on anything much.

*V/O Subchorionic haematoma. The aetiology of such haematomas is uncertain. Some authors have reported an association with thrombophilia and the presence of autoantibodies such as anti-cardiolipin. Foetal loss rates of twenty-five to fifty per cent have been described in some studies. In the largest review to-date, high rates of premature delivery were found.' *

Words foretelling our future? Signed off work to rest.

I can do little. I sit and crochet. Each stitch a moment of suspension.

Blankets made of love and hope.

The haematoma – now grown to over eight centimetres wide between the two babies and threatening the placentas.

V/O 'This is a pregnancy at risk.'
'You will still bleed, but you might be lucky and hold on to the babies.'

I cherish each minute holding you in case it's the last.

At seventeen weeks the blood stops.

The haematoma resolves, no sign on the scan.

* Loi K, Tan K. (2006) Massive pre-placental and subchorionic haematoma. Singapore Med J. Dec;47(12):1084-6.

Justine Bold @justinebold

But pregnancy loss is common right?

"But pregnancy loss is common, right?" The first time I had a loss, this was a common thing for people to say when I told them what happened.

They also say:
"It happens to a lot more people than you know"

"My friend had one and now she has four children! So, you'll be fine!"

"It can happen to people before they even realize they're pregnant"

"A lot of pregnancies end early"

"Don't worry, you can just get pregnant again"

"At least you got pregnant."

And the list goes on ... and none of these are helpful.

But people just don't understand. Yes, pregnancy loss is common, and, yes, I know I'm not the only one to ever experience it ... but it was new to me. And it hurt me. It hurt us. And everyone's experience is unique.

I always felt I had to justify that I ALSO did IVF to get pregnant – so it wasn't easy to even get a positive pregnancy. I'd fought like hell just for that.

Then I had a second loss after IVF. And guess what? It hurt just as much. And I was just as surprised. Just as broken. If not even more. Because now I've come to believe that it's the only possible outcome for my body.

And even when I didn't technically get pregnant, even when I had a failed transfer – it felt like a loss in ways that many people cannot understand. When a failed transfer happens, after a perfect embryo that we fought like hell for, prepared my body so long for, waited and waited for, is placed in exactly the right place, and it still doesn't want to hold on … it's devastating. Physically, pregnancy loss is harder, but emotionally, it's the same. They're both losses.

Pregnancy loss happens to about twenty-five per cent of women. And yes, many go on to have healthy children after, but some don't, and some have a recurrent loss (a much lower percentage), and no answers. But no matter what, there shouldn't be a competition in loss – it's ALL loss. And no statistics or personal stories can mend that pain.

Pregnancy loss is such a taboo subject – it makes people uncomfortable and sad so they'd rather just sugar-coat it and move on. And I know it's impossible to say the right thing, but it's not impossible to stop discounting people's traumas.

If someone shares a trauma with you, such as a pregnancy loss, it's okay to simply tell them that you're sorry – to say that it sucks and it's awful and that you're here for them.

Sometimes that's all we want to hear. And sometimes we just need to talk about it, and just know we won't be judged or criticized or questioned. We just want our trauma to be recognized and mourned, and accepted for what it is – loss! And that we need to grieve. And there's no timeline for that.

Alex @wheneverybodymatters

Pregnancy loss isn't talked about in society

When I had my first pregnancy loss, I didn't know what to expect. It never occurred to me that it would happen to me, nor did I think that it would happen a second time. Pregnancy loss isn't something that's talked about in society, let alone taught in schools. And because it's such a taboo subject, it leaves the person experiencing it with a sense of extreme shame and guilt.

If you're reading this and you've experienced one or more losses, I want you to know I am really sorry. You didn't do anything wrong and it wasn't your fault. You didn't lose your baby or babies because you ate something you shouldn't have, or drank too much or exercised too hard. Everything you're feeling is completely normal, even when you don't feel like it is. There is no right or wrong way to be or feel. I remember after my first pregnancy loss I had no idea of the amount of physical and emotional toll it would take on me. I was lucky enough to have a few weeks off work, but all I wanted to do was stay at home and sit on the sofa in front of the telly all day. I couldn't even bring myself to walk to the local shop, partly because I was so fatigued and partly because I just couldn't face the outside world.

Some days, grief will hit you out of the blue, and that's normal. Don't fight it or suppress it. Instead, on those days, acknowledge and honour your feelings and try to sit with it. In my early days of grief, I would often break down and sob uncontrollably and I couldn't understand why. I was so confused – what was wrong with me? I felt like I was losing my mind. I couldn't tell if what I was feeling was grief, anxiety, fear, guilt or shame. I know now that it was ALL of those things. It took another seven months for me to realise that I needed help. My husband Matt thinks I was in denial and maybe he's right. Or maybe I was so overwhelmed by all the different emotions, I just needed time to take it all in and process it.

After my second pregnancy loss, the following months went by in a haze. It felt unfair that the world around me carried on as if nothing happened, and even though I was back in my usual routine of commuting to work, pretending I was fine, (not many people knew I was pregnant at work, let alone had lost the baby), and commuting back home every day, I still felt incredibly sad and broken-hearted. My brain was in a constant fog, my heart heavy and all I could think about was the baby I'd lost. It was only when I searched the Miscarriage Association's website that I came across a pregnancy loss support group in West London. I plucked up the courage to attend, along with Matt. It was the first time we had spoken publicly about our losses in front of complete strangers, and it was such a relief to tell our story to others who had gone through a similar situation, and not feel judged in any way. I encourage you to reach out to those who have experienced the same heartache as you. Just being able to talk about your feelings and emotions to those that understand can make a huge difference.

If you think it will help to speak to a counsellor or therapist, seek one out. There are lots out there including a few charities that provide free counselling. The charity I used is called City Pregnancy and they provide up to ten free sessions for those working and living in and around London in the UK. I had no prior experience of counselling, and like a lot of people, felt ashamed that I needed help. Once I got over that, I tried to keep an open mind and went with it. It was the single best thing I did for myself and my mental health. Therapy isn't for everyone and it's not going to 'cure' you, but what it will do is provide a safe space for you to express your fears and process your thoughts, which will support your healing process.

Not everyone will understand what you're going through and not every person will be able to empathise and that's OK, because we're all built very differently. Find those you can confide in who won't pass judgement and hold those people close to you. They will be the ones you'll need to lean on in those dark moments when you're struggling to face the world. Aside from the comfort of your friends and family, there is a wonderfully supportive and compassionate community tucked away in a corner of Instagram. I was lucky enough to find it via one of the (many) podcasts I listened to back in my early days of grief, and it has been a real lifesaver for which I'll always be grateful. These women and men just 'get it'. We each may be on different journeys, but we all share the same end goal. You can engage with the community as much or as little as you want – you can even do this via an anonymous account. It's completely up to you how you want to make use of it, but know that if you ever want to rant, moan or need some comforting words, we are there for you.

If, like me, you lost your baby in the first trimester, please don't think that your baby matters any less than a baby that died much later. Unfortunately, it's very common for women to feel like they shouldn't complain 'too much.' It doesn't matter whether your baby died at two weeks or forty weeks, it's still heart-breaking because it was everything you had ever hoped and longed for. Don't feel like you shouldn't grieve because someone else had it 'harder,' or because it's been five years so 'why am I not over it by now?'

It doesn't help when society tells us that we shouldn't announce our pregnancy before the twelve-week scan. Neither is it helpful that the medical world is still so far behind when it comes to providing the right support and care for those who have an early pregnancy loss, because it's 'so common.' This just adds to the shame.

It will take time to process your grief and to heal. And that's ok. Take each day as it comes and don't feel like you have to 'get over it,' because like for many of us, you never will. You just become better at dealing with it. Losing a baby changes you. It changes your outlook on life. It's easy to be really hard on yourself (I do it all the time), but in those moments, ask yourself, if this was your friend, what would you say to them?

Despite the nightmare you're going through, you will come out the other side, and there is light at the end of the tunnel. I, for one, have learnt so much about myself through therapy and as a result of my losses, have become more empathetic and less judgmental of others, (you never know what pain someone else is hiding). My husband and I are the closest we've ever been. There have been days where we've really struggled but we've learnt to communicate better with each other, and respect that we both grieve very differently.

I wish I had someone to tell me all of these things when I went through my pregnancy losses, but I take some comfort that I'm able to offer these words to you now. Please know that however lonely and isolated you're feeling, you are not alone and there is a wonderful Instagram community out there to support you and be there for you.

Yuen Kwan Li @over40_tryingforababy

I'm pregnant but I've lost it

2017 was meant to be a very different beginning for my husband and I, but it was the month that changed the course of our lives. Mid-February we went in for what was meant to be a ten-week ultrasound, only to have all my worst fears become reality.

"I'm sorry there's no heartbeat" ... that can't be it, it just can't be. I thought the technician must have made a mistake and I wanted them to keep checking until they found it beating again. My heart was pounding, I couldn't swallow, I was breathing fast, my mind going a million miles an hour with all the possibilities. My world froze.

The technician left the room to get someone more senior and I remember turning to my husband in shock, but at the same time hopeful that when they returned, they'd find a way to hear the heartbeat.

"I'm sorry" they said after doing the scan again. I remember the disbelief. I turned to my husband again but this time I broke down and cried ... a heaving, heart-breaking, soul-shattering wail. My whole world collapsed as my husband held me.

We rang the doctor's surgery from the ultrasound clinic and made a beeline for the surgery, trying to avoid anyone who might want to stop and talk to us. The doctor sat us down and I remember her looking at me and shedding tears too. She told me what to expect over the coming days and weeks as my body would naturally let go of our baby.

We went to my mums to tell her the news and she also broke down. We all cried together as a family, and I felt numb. I didn't have any strength left in me at that stage.

Once at home, it didn't take long for my body to start losing the pregnancy, and I have never felt so alone. I had my husband, my mum and my in-laws, but I didn't know anyone who'd been through it to ask for help.

We were googling the symptoms I was experiencing as they weren't what the doctor had said to expect. I was fainting, had horrid cramps, which I later found out were contractions, and at one stage I called my mum and said, "I'm going to die." I ended up being rushed to our nearest hospital and receiving surgery to have a D&C.

You barely feel like you can get over the trauma when you realise that you have to tell people what's happening in your new world. The hardest words you'll ever have to say are: "I'm pregnant but I've lost the baby." I'm so grateful now for my parents and in-laws support after telling them I was pregnant from the start, and didn't have to explain anything to them. Honestly, why should we feel we have to wait the thirteen weeks to tell anyone!

I sat in my car to call my boss at work. I thought I was composed and able to tell them what had happened, but as soon as I uttered those words, I was crying uncontrollably. I had to take a deep breath and start again. I didn't expect it to be so hard, but saying those few words is so emotional.

It's honestly one of the hardest and emotional composition of words you will have to say in your life. They are so heart-wrenching and personal. All I wanted at this time was someone to listen objectively or let me cry, vent, or just sit and be numb. It's only human to want to make sense of it all and have answers to the unanswerable. Most of the time, it's just mother nature doing her thing, and unfortunately, we must try and move on without knowing why. And we can move forward without forgetting about our angel babies.

It's important to focus on yourself at this time – be selfish, set boundaries, do whatever's necessary to heal. You're grieving so allow that to happen. This isn't a time to try and please others. You need to be gentle on yourself – you're doing the best you can considering what's happened.

Sharna Southan @sharnasouthan_coaching

Healing after ectopic pregnancy loss

I remember it all so clearly. It was our first prenatal scan and we were convinced that this would finally be the baby that stayed with us. My husband and I anxiously awaited good news from our doctor. Instead, what we heard were the dreaded words, "There's nothing in your uterus. I'm concerned that it's an ectopic pregnancy."

I'll never forget how shattering it was. Those words were uttered in such a matter-of-fact manner that it completely crushed my heart. A follow-up scan confirmed that the foetus was implanted in my right fallopian tube instead of my uterus, my tube was ruptured, and I was bleeding internally. The most heart-breaking thing was seeing our baby's heartbeat flickering on the monitor as if they were doing all they could to thrive, and then being told that my pregnancy was not viable and that I was at risk of losing my own life too. As a result, I ended up having emergency surgery (a laparoscopic salpingectomy), and lost both my baby and my right fallopian tube.

The surgery was fast. I was discharged from hospital a day later, but when the dust of this frightening and painful whirlwind settled, I was left bereft. I've found that little prepares you for the aftermath of going through a fate you'd hoped would never happen. I'd naively thought I understood loss because of my previous pregnancy losses, and I'd half expected that this time it would be somewhat easier for me to endure.

I soon learned how wrong I was on both accounts. It was completely bewildering to discover how different experiencing an ectopic pregnancy was from this loss, how much more jarring and devastating it felt. An already difficult emotional healing process now required me to come to terms with the added trauma of emergency surgery, and a more complicated physical recovery before I could even consider trying to conceive again. It also meant getting to grips with an uncertain future now that I had only one remaining fallopian tube and a ten per cent higher chance of having another ectopic pregnancy.

The journey to healing and recovery

The initial weeks post-surgery were the hardest I've had to live through. It scared me how low I felt, and I was so afraid that I'd never get over the debilitating sadness that permeated everything. Needless to say, recovery after my ectopic pregnancy loss was a slow and challenging journey. Needless to say, recovery after my ectopic pregnancy loss was a slow and challenging journey. I needed to consciously nurture myself and create space for emotional processing. Simply practicing mindfulness, meditation and other relaxation therapies helped me to build my coping skills and resilience. I created space to grieve. My husband and I did a grief release ceremony to honour and say goodbye to our baby. This was a deeply cathartic experience that gave us both a sense of closure. I also reached out for emotional assistance, went for healing sessions and found supportive people to talk to as I worked through my depression. Having an incredible support system to lean on was a profound saving grace during that time. Having an incredible support system to lean on was a profound saving grace during that time. The emotional fallout after a pregnancy loss can be so isolating, so if you feel overwhelmed by all that you're going through, it's so important to lean on your support system. Accept help when you need it. Go for counselling if necessary. Also, consider joining a support group. Being in a community with other women who share similar experiences to yours is healing, and helps you feel less alone in your struggles.

As the weeks went by, the layers of depression slowly began to lift and I found it a little easier to breathe through the heaviness. Getting out of bed in the morning became less of a struggle, and the days seemed less daunting as I felt more able to tackle everyday tasks again. With time, I felt that the worst was behind me and that I'd come through something momentous, but also somewhat stunned at the level of inner strength I'd unearthed within myself.

PTSD and anxiety

Several months later when we'd received the go-ahead to try and conceive again, I encountered another hurdle that I'd not experienced with previous pregnancy losses. I was overcome by bouts of anxiety and unexpected panic attacks. At first, it felt misplaced and came seemingly from nowhere because I couldn't pinpoint it to anything specific. Suddenly, ordinary situations felt overwhelmingly stressful and my body would shut down because I couldn't breathe properly. It took me several weeks to recognize that I was experiencing some degree of post-traumatic stress disorder (PTSD), most likely triggered when I got back to trying to conceive.

The unfortunate reality is that when you've experienced pregnancy loss, (especially more than once), it becomes difficult to trust in your body's ability to conceive and carry a healthy pregnancy to term. There is always the fear that it will happen again. Every twitch, sensation or dull ache becomes a trigger. Knowing that the ectopic was life-threatening made it hard to trust that I was safe or healthy. It was a catch-22 situation. I feared not being able to get pregnant again and at the same time, I feared the possibility of becoming pregnant only to experience another loss. I struggled with intimacy because I was afraid that if I conceived too soon, I would have another ectopic pregnancy. I guess once you've experienced the worst-case scenario, your mind always assumes that it will happen again, fearful of reliving the same trauma, only not being able to survive it all this time around, so you remain in fight-or-flight mode; tense, anxious and mistrusting.

Once more, I had to take steps to support my mental and emotional wellbeing and seek out the right kind of assistance. I gave myself more time to understand my triggers and to work through them. Along with doing the 'inner' emotional work and releasing my physical tension, a key focus was rebuilding my trust in my body, as well as my confidence in my ability to conceive and have a healthy full-term pregnancy. It also put my mind at ease to focus more on the ninety per cent chance that the baby will implant in the right place and that I will have a healthy normal pregnancy next time around, rather than the ten per cent chance of having another ectopic pregnancy.

In closing, I'll say that although it hasn't been an easy ride, I am cognizant of the profound lessons I've gained. I've seen that even with the bad, there's room to learn and grow. To anyone who's navigating recovery after ectopic pregnancy loss, know that you're not alone. You're doing the best that you can, so be extra kind and gentle with yourself. And remember, sometimes healing is a slow process – one breath at a time, one step at a time, one day at a time. And most importantly, remember to reach out for help if you're feeling overwhelmed. Not everyone will understand or be sympathetic to your experiences – it's therefore important to surround yourself with a few positive, reliable people who you'll be able to lean on when needed.

Jodi Sky Rogers @thefertilemoon

Ten things to remember when you're experiencing pregnancy loss

This wasn't your fault. When I had my first pregnancy loss, instantly, I thought of the extra cup of coffee that I'd had the week before. The guilt that we, as women feel after pregnancy loss, is something that only those who've been through it understand. It's so important to know that nothing you did caused your loss.

You may think that now you have to start over, but that's not true. Those first few weeks of pregnancy feel like they'll last forever, and all you want is to reach the second trimester so you can tell the world that you're now pregnant. When you learn that you're losing a baby, it's common to feel like you're starting from square one, but that's not how it works. Your body has conceived and held life, no matter how short.

Despite what you believe, you're not broken. Your body served as the perfect home and cared for that life as long as it was given the opportunity. There's absolutely nothing BROKEN about you.

Remember that you're recovering and give yourself time to do that. After a pregnancy loss, it's sometimes hard to remember that you're recovering, because it's treated differently than a standard postpartum period in the eyes of others. Allow yourself to recover, rest, and heal. There are no guidelines for emotional or physical recovery. Be patient with yourself.

Your feelings are valid (no matter what they may be). Everyone grieves differently and that's okay. No matter if you're sad, angry or confused – all emotions are valid and you have every right to feel however you feel.

Just because you didn't get the chance to bring home and hold this baby in your arms, doesn't mean that you never will. A baby that's conceived after pregnancy loss is referred to as a RAINBOW BABY, so believe that you'll meet your rainbow. Losing one baby doesn't mean that you'll lose all of them.

It's up to you to choose if you would like to share the news of your pregnancy. A lot of people wait until twelve plus weeks of pregnancy to share the news with family and friends, so if they experience a loss before then, others don't know what they're going through. Don't be afraid to share this news but also, don't be afraid to keep it to yourself. At the end of the day, it's your decision.

Drink the coffee, a glass of wine, or a caffeinated soda. A common emotion after pregnancy loss is GUILT, especially when you start doing things you wouldn't have done while pregnant. Maybe it's a meal that you wouldn't eat while pregnant or drinking a few glasses of wine. Be kind to yourself, you deserve a treat.

Speak up and ask for help if you need physical, mental, or emotional support. There's an unnecessary stigma that surrounds pregnancy loss and talking about our fertility in general. Don't let that make you feel like you have to struggle in private. There are resources available to you no matter where you are in your journey or grief. Ask for help.

Most importantly, remember that you are strong, capable, and brave. You will get through this. There are times when you'll wonder how you'll dig yourself out of your grief, or you'll wonder if the weight of your loss will ever lighten, but I promise, it will.

Arden Cartrette @ardenmcartrette

Wave of light to commemorate all babies who
sadly died too soon

Grief never leaves us completely

If you've suffered a pregnancy loss, then you'll understand the devastation that takes over your world – the confusion of wondering what happened to your baby or why your body failed you. You wanted that baby more than anything in the world and somehow that dream was ruined. Over time, you begin to heal and pray you'll get pregnant again, but fear and guilt can take over. You may feel you're not honoring your lost baby if you have another. You might wonder how you'll ever be brave enough to try again.

I'd like to share my story in the hope of providing support, a virtual hug, and some guidance on how to manage the pain and move forward. First, I'd like to say how sorry I am for your loss and that it's NOT your fault. I promise you, it's never your fault. Here's my story of our four losses and our miracle baby that I thought would never happen.

My husband and I met in 2008, during my very first shift as a traveling nurse in Phoenix, Arizona. We immediately hit it off and became good friends. We had a lot of fun and enjoyed being around each other but we were never going to date! But our love was inevitable and we couldn't fight our feelings any longer and after six months we began our lives together.

We lived a very adventurous existence, travelling as much as we could. We learned to mountain bike, salsa dance, surf, wakeboard, snowboard and explored many different beautiful places. I was twenty-eight and my partner was thirty-one, but we didn't think we'd have any issues starting a family, like most people, I suppose.

In 2012, I had a pregnancy loss; we didn't even know I was pregnant! I was confused and deeply sad. I was about to start a new job that week and my husband and I weren't yet married, so, I believed God knew what was best for us and that this was simply not our time to start a family.

A year later, we got married in Sedona, Arizona. It was a

wonderful, magical day. Five months into our marriage we found out we were pregnant! It was perfect timing so this time it had to be right, didn't it? I even did a cute "surprise" your husband event and we imagined how our lives would be with a baby who'd then become a child, and then a teenager. We even had a name picked out if the baby was a girl.

Unfortunately, this pregnancy also ended in pregnancy loss at seven weeks. This time, we were devastated. I remember seeing the blood and rushing to the doctor in a panic, praying that I wasn't losing our baby, that somehow, we'd be OK. When I sat in the doctor's office waiting, I just knew it wasn't going to be OK. My body ached, my mind was spinning and I felt broken. How could this be happening?

I didn't know many people who'd gone through this and I hadn't spoken much about my first loss, so I wasn't sure how to grieve. Because of this, I didn't have anyone else to talk to; I felt very alone and wasn't sure how to deal with my feelings.

I was involved in a one-hundred-mile bike race for charity two weeks after my pregnancy loss, but I was only able to complete fifty miles as I was unable to keep up with my group. I was riding alone for most of the race with tears streaming down my face. I felt as if I had no one and everything was completely surreal.

After having my second pregnancy loss, I thought there must be something wrong with me so I began seeing a different OB (Obstetrician). Shortly after, when medications and timed intercourse weren't working either, I was diagnosed with 'undiagnosed recurrent pregnancy loss.' Super helpful, right? And so began my official fertility journey.

We met an incredible fertility specialist who listened, sympathised, and told me he could help me get pregnant and carry my baby to full term. Oh, my goodness … to hear those words … to hear someone believe in you, that you will become a mom. I was elated and scared but so ready to start a family with my loving husband.

Over the next few months my life was consumed with doctor's appointments, injections, diet changes, detoxing my household and my body, decreasing my stress, and taking tons of supplements and hormones. All of these steps were part of the process to have my dream baby and I poured my entire self into all of it, feeling relieved that some of it was in my control. I was determined, and thought that if I did everything 'right' I would finally become a mom.

After many months we were ready, physically and emotionally, to take the next big step – IUI (Intrauterine insemination). We knew the odds of getting pregnant on the first IUI treatment were low, but we couldn't help but be hopeful. Our results came in and I was pregnant! I was shocked but excited. I planned a special way to surprise my husband and we fell in love all over again.

However, after several weeks, the baby was determined to be 'not viable' and the harsh reality sank in again. I was so upset and couldn't believe it was happening. We'd done everything right and beaten the odds. To top it all, this was the only appointment my husband ever missed, just a routine visit for IV (intravenous) meds. I wasn't supposed to get the lab test until later that day when I was home with him. I had to drive the one-hour trip alone and I was heartbroken. I also hadn't had the actual pregnancy loss yet, so my body was still showing signs I was pregnant. It was such a mind f*ck.

The worst part was feeling betrayed by my body. Thirteen weeks later, I still hadn't released our baby and knowing they weren't alive anymore, I couldn't carry on like this. We went to our doctor's again and I was given 'pills' to take as our worst nightmare unfolded several hours later.

I've never experienced so much physical and mental pain in my entire life. I couldn't walk. There was blood everywhere. My body felt like it was being ripped in half. It was the absolute worst experience of my life. My husband was also really sick at the time, but despite being weak he carried me to and from the bed to the bathroom so many times over several days.

He was so strong for me, physically and emotionally. I will never forget the love I felt from him. I can't describe the way this type of loss brought us together. It was raw, ugly, and so real.

I know everyone responds in their own way to a pregnancy loss but I was shaken to my core. I was no longer able to say 'it wasn't meant to be.' It was a very dark time. I share these details not only to shed light on the devastation that happens with pregnancy loss, but also to share some insight as to why immense fear builds up for those who've suffered a single loss or recurrent losses.

After our third pregnancy loss, when I knew that I'd done everything 'right' and still the efforts didn't produce our miracle baby, I was done. I thought there was no way I was ever going to try again. How could I possibly go through this pain over and over? But something inside of me wasn't ready to give up completely. I knew I had to begin some serious inner work and start healing.

Over the next few months, I researched grieving and 'recurrent pregnancy loss.' I realized all three losses had created intense grief and I needed time to feel that pain and understand my love for our babies. I've learnt that grief never leaves us completely. It's not a process you go through and then complete. It's something that's part of you because you loved this new being. But you can learn to live with grief and understand that it doesn't have to consume you.

One of the most powerful resources I found to help with my fear and anxiety was a book entitled The Miracle of Mindfulness: An Introduction to the Practice of Meditation by Thich Nhat Hanh. Like many people, I struggle with traditional meditating, but what I loved about this book was that it helped me remain in the present.

I used simple breathing exercises several times a week when the fear escalated. Thich Nhat Hanh states that "whenever your mind becomes scattered, use your breath as the means to take hold of your thoughts again". Here's an example of how he walks you through an effective way to remain present while breathing and connecting your body to your thoughts.

Take hold of your breath in the following manner: "Be ever mindful as you breathe in and mindful as you breathe out. Breathing in a long breath, think, 'I am breathing in a long breath.' Breathing out a long breath, think, 'I am breathing out a long breath.' Breathing in a short breath, think, 'I am breathing in a short breath.' Breathing out a short breath, think, 'I am breathing out a short breath.'

Performing this way of breathing allows you to only focus on one thing; your breath. You can no longer fill your head with a million fearful thoughts. I found this to be a little awkward at first, but soon I no longer had to think about the words. When my heart raced or I felt panicky or sad, I would begin breathing like this and immediately my body and mind would become calm.

During this time, I realized that I never acknowledged the grief for my babies was very real. We never had a ceremony, we didn't name them, and we barely told anyone. A very dear friend of mine gave me a beautiful Angel Sweet Pea necklace. When I opened the box, I gasped. Inside was this necklace with three little pearls in a pea pod that represented my three babies. This was the first tangible item I had to represent my little angels. Wearing this necklace meant I could rub the pearls and feel a connection to my babies when I felt scared of trying again. Whether you wear a necklace, create a memory box, have a ceremony, name your baby or whatever feels right for you, it's so important to acknowledge the loss of your baby and truly grieve the life you carried.

During this process of healing, I also realized that I needed to do something to stop me feeling lost and depressed all the time – something to make me dig deep, to find some peace, even if I didn't always want to. I was never into keeping a journal, but I found a few that were written for pregnancy loss or child loss which helped me to refocus my negative energy and begin healing. I needed prompts but also wanted free space to just write down my feelings on my worst days where I'd pour my heart out. It was emotionally raw but also incredibly therapeutic.

If you're thinking this isn't for you, I encourage you to take a chance; try journaling for one week. You may be surprised at how impactful writing down your thoughts and painful emotions can be.

After I spent this precious time focusing on healing, we decided to try IUI again. This time we were pregnant with twins! Wow, what a miracle. We couldn't believe it and all my symptoms felt different this time. However, at thirteen weeks one of our baby's heart stopped beating. It was quite a difficult loss because we were so happy, we had one healthy baby, but equally devastated we'd lost yet another, and especially a twin. But we had a healthy baby girl, and I'm so thankful every day that I didn't give up and learnt how to heal after so much tragedy.

Wherever you are in your journey, I know it's hard and terrifying. I've provided a few ideas that truly helped me find my courage and take the next step forward. Dig deep and discover what's holding you back. Write down your thoughts, acknowledge those fears and conquer them head-on. Reach out to those who've gone through the same journey and would love to support you. You never know what could be just around the corner. It could be a beautiful rainbow baby.

Jackie Figueras @jackiefigueras

At least you know you can get pregnant

"At least you know you can get pregnant" – that's what a female family member said to me. Brene Brown, a Professor and Researcher in Shame and Vulnerability produced a short video explaining empathy versus sympathy:

The fox said she had a 'miscarriage', the gazelle replied: "At least you know you can get pregnant."

Empathy never starts with "At least!"

People really don't know what to say and many don't understand. People don't see a pregnancy loss as the loss of a child, the loss of a baby, of a potential human being, the loss of future and hope. I didn't at first...

In the beginning, I was carrying a bunch of cells, an embryo, not viable outside the womb. It wasn't until I read a book and attended sessions with Child Bereavement UK that my perspective changed. We never named our kids, too early to know their genders, although now we want to commemorate them. My husband and I have lost three potential human beings with all their lives ahead of them – three babies that we won't be able to cuddle and nurture, three kids that won't go to school.

Each of my three pregnancy losses have been physically different, although all have mentally scarred and tormented my husband and I. All occurred in the first trimester when it's not really spoken about or understood. There's no recognition, no funeral, no ceremony, and most people don't even know someone is going through it. It's still taboo – death in general is, despite the stats.

Our first pregnancy loss was from a natural pregnancy in 2015. I started bleeding at work and went straight to St Thomas' Early Pregnancy & Gynae Unit (EPAGU). I'd been told about them as you don't need a GP referral. It's a nurse-led unit and all of the team are phenomenal, very kind and caring. I've used their services more than anywhere else, as they're especially clued up and understanding.

I chose to take tablets to speed the process along. It's hard to know when it's going to pass – the bleeding lasts for days and the womb lining and bits of pregnancy tissue are either in your knickers or drop into the toilet. It's physically uncomfortable, the cramping and the pain, and mentally exhausting.

Our second pregnancy was also natural after lots of fertility treatment had failed. The bleeding started again. This time I contacted my GP who referred me to the Early Pregnancy Unit at my local hospital. I went several times and although the embryo had grown, the nurse had never heard or seen a heartbeat, yet allowed me to go on for eleven weeks. She should have called in a gynaecologist much sooner. I went straight back to St Thomas' and chose to have it removed surgically and then tested. Despite having a local anaesthetic, it was still incredibly painful and lasted longer than it was supposed to, so they had to call in a senior gynaecologist. Randomly I remember coloured fairy lights in the ceiling. I saw the embryo this time. It felt strange. I had the choice to keep it or have it disposed of. I chose the latter. I didn't even consult my husband.

After seeing various gynaecologists privately, we were recommended to use a donor, so our third pregnancy was after using a donor egg and sperm. I had our third pregnancy loss and the baby was removed surgically with a general anaesthetic in the outpatients at St Thomas'. When I came round the female gynaecologist barely acknowledged me, didn't introduce herself and was really rude. I felt alone and isolated. A female nurse who wheeled me round to the recovery suite chatted to a male nurse, telling him she'd had a baby and then had the insensitive audacity to look at me and say "Don't worry, it'll happen to you." I was completely gob-smacked. I told her that she had no idea what I'd been through and that I'd been trying for years. She replied that she'd tried for even longer. I had just had another baby removed and it appeared as if the nurse was competing with me. I made a formal complaint about both staff members and was advised that training from the EPAGU (Early Pregnancy and Acute Gynaecology Unit) team was going to be booked for all nursing staff. I hope it happened.

I've had lots of investigations these past seven years of trying to have a family, seen lots of gynaecologists and a Recurrent Miscarriage Specialist. Multiple issues have been found including being diagnosed with Hashimoto's Thyroiditis, heterozygous factor V Leiden, Lupus anticoagulant and an arcuate (heart-shaped) uterus, which has since been operated on.

My husband and I attended a Miscarriage Association support group and met a woman who'd been on Heparin. When she experienced her pregnancy loss, both she and her husband said it was like a bloodbath as her blood was so thin. I now have to take Heparin and visualise a 'Carrie-esque' scenario like the movie, if I end up losing my baby again.

I still don't have a baby or child of my own, and I don't know if I ever will. Have I been a Mum though? Well, I've carried three potential babies, but in the eyes of the law, no, I'm not. It's only been since my husband and I had a year's bereavement counselling and a break from trying to get pregnant, that I want to fully acknowledge our three babies. We'd like to get a water feature with three channels to have in our garden, to remember the three lives that weren't meant to be.

Lauren Juggler-Crook

Shattered dreams after a 'missed miscarriage'

We walked into hospital that day with so much joy, hope and excitement. Little did we know that it was also going to be the day our lives changed forever. Just seventeen days before we got married, we found out at our twelve-week scan that we'd lost our precious baby – we had what's termed a 'missed miscarriage', and it's when a baby has died in the womb, but the mother hasn't had any symptoms, such as bleeding or pain. Any type of pregnancy loss can cause shock, but a 'missed miscarriage' can be particularly difficult because of the lack of symptoms.

Everything had changed. We weren't who we were before. Our hearts were broken and our dreams shattered. I also felt like I'd let my family down too. The worst thing is having no answers and no reason as to why it happened. We were just told the statistics of one in four and somehow that's supposed to make you feel better, as if it's normal. It feels like you're told to deal with it because you're not the only one even though it feels like you are. It's a very lonely experience unless you talk to other women who've also been through it. I will never get the image out of my head of our baby on the monitor. I will be forever terrified of scans.

However, we're determined to carry on and have our rainbow baby one day. A rainbow baby is a name coined for a healthy baby born after a pregnancy loss, infant loss, stillbirth or neonatal death. If there's any advice I'd give to anyone who's gone through this, it's not to blame yourself – you did everything you could. Stay strong and keep telling yourself there will be light at the end of the tunnel. Although you'll never forget the trauma you've been through, it does get easier.

Katy Jenkins @thejstartshere & ivf_got_this_uk

91

I wasn't ready for the miracle to end

I woke up, showered and got ready for work as normal. I went to the bathroom before I left and noticed I was bleeding. I knew immediately what was happening but I didn't want to believe it. It had only been a few days before that I'd had my positive pregnancy test and enjoyed four days of sharing this wonderful, magical secret with my husband. We'd been trying for the best part of a year, so to be pregnant seemed like a miracle. And I wasn't ready for that miracle to end.

I sent my husband off to work with a "don't worry, I'm sure it's nothing" whilst I called the GP who instantly booked me in to see her. She took my blood pressure and then booked me in for a scan at the hospital – but that was still a week away. I was told to go home but if the bleeding got heavier or if I was in pain, I should go to A&E (Accident & Emergency).

I went home and sat on my sofa in disbelief. Did I really have to sit at home waiting for the inevitable to happen? Was there nothing I could do? An hour later, the bleeding became heavier – so heavy in fact, it was a struggle to control it, so I ended up sitting on the loo rather than going through ten sanitary pads. It was at this point that I decided to head to hospital. My sister had been staying with us so I ended up telling her everything. It was heart-breaking to see the joy on her face but then her eyes well up when I told her I might be losing my longed-for baby.

I thought I knew what would happen when I arrived at the hospital as this was an emergency, so I expected to be rushed through to have a scan immediately. However, once there, I had to fill out a form at reception and then wait with my sister in A&E with lots of other people with various ailments. So that's what we did for three hours! During this time my sister did her best to distract me, but the bleeding became heavier, which involved visiting the bathroom every five minutes. Then a stabbing pain ripped through my stomach. I staggered up from my chair and asked reception how long it might be before I saw someone, as I was feeling uncomfortable and upset. The lady looked sympathetic and said she'd give me some paracetamol while I waited. The pain was like a cramping period pain but a lot worse. I had to hug my knees to ease it. I tried to keep control of my emotions as I didn't want to break down in front of my younger sister, and a room full of people.

Eventually, a female doctor beckoned me into a room. I went through everything that had happened and she took my blood pressure, felt my tummy, and then booked me in for an 'urgent' scan. Unfortunately, the scan was the same one a whole week away. I was told yet again to go home, take painkillers and rest. Seeing the anguish in my eyes she said, "Don't worry, you're still young, you'll have another one."

"But I want THIS one," I said as I wandered out of the room in a daze. My sister and I drove home and sat on the sofa in silence. The full reality of what was happening hit me and under my sister's care, I wept continually until I fell asleep.

A week later I went back for my scan at the maternity ward. I had to walk through a sea of pregnant ladies in various stages of their pregnancies probably going for their twelve and twenty-week scans, and then I got taken into a quiet room at the back with a few chairs, some magazines and a box of tissues. This was the room for people like me who'd lost their baby.

It was over pretty quick. The midwife explained that I'd had a 'full miscarriage' which meant I wouldn't need surgery. "That's good I suppose," was all I could say. I felt so empty, numb and alone. Nobody at that moment could understand exactly how I felt, no matter how much they supported me and said kind things.

Lianne Baker

We'd seen the heartbeat

When we started IVF (in-vitro fertilization), we thought it meant a guaranteed result. We'd go through the process, the shots, the hormones, but then we'd get to choose the gender of our baby and become pregnant a few months later! But that wasn't the case. It took us seven transfers and four egg retrievals to get to what was considered a 'safe pregnancy week.' – which is where I am as I write this. So, let's just say, it hasn't been a walk in the park over the past three years.

In December 2018, after my third transfer and my third egg retrieval, we were pregnant. We were elated! While we didn't PGS (pre-implantation genetic screening*) test the embryo, we figured, since it hung on and we became pregnant, it must be a healthy embryo. Never in my wildest dreams did I think something could go wrong.

We went into the fertility center on what was supposed to be our 'graduation day;' week eight. As the doctor began the intravaginal ultrasound, he was quiet. He was usually quiet, but this time, more so. "It doesn't look good: the baby has stopped growing."

My heart sank and all I could do was sob and hold onto Nick's arm asking why and how could this happen. We'd only just seen the heartbeat ten days ago! The doctor and the nurse left the room while I slowly got dressed. I remember thinking, now what? How can we just go back to being 'normal?' How can we move on with our life? How are we going to tell our seven-year-old twin daughters, since we'd already told them the good news? I remember it like it was yesterday. It was the hardest day of my life.

I felt so alone as if something was wrong with me. How could I be so naïve to think everything would be OK? How could this happen after all we'd already been through?

That night we told the girls. They were sobbing and that made everything so much worse. I felt like the worst mom. I questioned why we'd told them so early on?

The next few days were hard. I had to go back to business as usual after planning my entire life around this new pregnancy. We'd even booked a baby moon.

The next few months were physically hard. I bled the entire time. I had to take two Misoprostol pills to help my body to pass all the tissue. But after almost three months, the doctor still found tissue in my uterus, and I ended up having a D&C anyway. That was hard to hear. But in a way, it was finally the closure I needed. The only way to move on and be able to try again.

Looking back, I never in a million years thought I'd be having a pregnancy loss. I never thought it would take this long to get pregnant and I certainly never thought I'd be documenting it all. But here I am, wanting to share because it happens to so many of us!

It's so unbelievably common and yet no one talks about it. I hope that my story makes just one person feel less alone, because we're not alone, and sometimes things happen and it's not our fault!

*PGS was replaced in 2019 with Preimplantation Genetic Testing or PGT, and there are three categories of tests – PGT-A, PGT-M and PFT-SR.

Erin @mybeautifulblunder

It wasn't an ectopic

Based on the blog: 'My first miscarriage'

Honestly, it was a faint line. A very faint line. But it was my first and I was beyond thrilled to see it. We'd been trying for about ten months and I was one week late for my period when I tested. The line was so faint that my husband wasn't convinced and suggested we test again before calling the doctor.

We went hiking the next day with friends and I remember being so happy about our little secret, but also worried about not overdoing it with the exercise or getting dehydrated. I hiked slowly, drank lots of water, and my husband kept telling me to stop grinning and holding my belly so our friends wouldn't suspect.

I waited a few days and tested again. I couldn't see a line. But my period hadn't arrived and I was cramping on the right side of my stomach around the area of my ovary, so I called the doctor anyway. They brought me in and did an ultrasound. I had a closed cervix! I was pregnant! I'd never been pregnant before and I was worried that I couldn't fall naturally, so I was thrilled. They congratulated me and told me not to worry about the pain on my right side, that they could see the cyst that released the egg was on the right ovary, and that was probably what the cramping was from. They weren't worried about not being able to see other things, because, after all, I was barely five weeks pregnant.

I was going to my regular Obstetrician (OB), so they didn't get the blood test results that day. I got a call a few days later from the nurse saying my hCG (human chorionic gonadotrophin hormone or pregnancy hormone), was thirty-three, so on the low side, but not to worry because it was still early. But every home pregnancy test I'd taken was negative. My right side was still really hurting and I'd been spending a lot of time with Dr Google. My husband and I were both worried about an ectopic, and why the hCG wasn't rising and I wasn't testing positive with a home pregnancy test.

The nurse told me to go straight to ER if I got dizzy, lightheaded, or had intense pain on my side. "Intense pain on my side?" I asked. "I thought we ruled out an ectopic with the scan." She said it was still possible, so they wanted to monitor me carefully.

I don't know why they didn't have me come back for a second hCG. Maybe it was because I didn't have a history of pregnancy loss. The Friday before when I was six weeks pregnant, I felt lightheaded and weak at work. I called the doctor and they told me to go straight to ER. I told my boss what was happening and she said, "Don't worry, I'm sure you and little peanut are just fine! Everyone gets lightheaded the first trimester."

At the ER they took my blood and did another ultrasound. There it was, no heartbeat yet, but a little sac right there in the uterus! On my smartphone, I turned once again to Dr Google to double-check that you couldn't have a sac AND an ectopic. I found a study that showed that though it was technically possible to have a 'pseudo sac' in the uterus, it was highly unlikely. I was reassured and we were so excited. We started brainstorming baby names while waiting to see the doctor. For twenty or so beautiful minutes we truly believed we were going to have a baby.

The doctor came in but wasn't smiling like we were. My hCG was thirty. Not only had it not doubled, it had also dropped lower. He told us the pregnancy was probably going to end soon, saying something about a 'blighted ovum.' They sent us home.

We prayed for a miracle for twenty-four hours until the cramps and the bleeding hit. I called my OB and they said to take Ibuprofen and come in on Monday to be checked. I spent the weekend bleeding, crying, and cuddled up with a heat pack and our cat. I passed a lot of large clots so I knew it was truly over.

On Monday I went into the OB for a scan. They said it was, "to ensure there's nothing left over." First, they gave me a Rhogam shot in case the embryo's heart was already pumping blood, since I have a negative blood type and my husband was positive.

Then I had the scan. At first, the tech thought things looked fine as nothing was left in the uterus. Then she got concerned as it looked like there might be bleeding in the tube. We waited to see the doctor. He said we had to go to ER immediately, again.

I protested. "I've already passed multiple large clots, I don't have any pain on the side anymore, are you SURE you can see bleeding in the tube?" He said he couldn't be sure, but to be on the safe side I needed to go to ER. Only there could I get the results of an hCG test immediately rather than waiting for days if the OB did it. I went with a printout of the scan.

At the ER they took my blood and we waited for the doctor, who came in with forms for us to sign. I needed emergency surgery for an ectopic pregnancy.

"BUT aren't we going to wait for the hCG levels to come back?"

"No, we can't waste time.'

"BUT ... I feel FINE, can't you just monitor me closely and get me ready to go into surgery if I tank?"

"No, we can't risk your life by waiting."

"BUT the sac was IN THE UTERUS. We saw it on the scan!"

"We haven't seen that scan. We can't risk it."

It was the same ER I'd been to earlier that week. I still don't understand why they couldn't see the earlier scan.

"BUT I PASSED HUGE CLOTS ALL WEEKEND."

"Did you save the tissue?"

"No!"

We agreed and called the hospital priest who gave me the Blessing of the Sick and said a prayer for my Fallopian tubes, as there was a risk I might lose one during surgery. Catholics really get this kind of stuff.

I'd been awake from the surgery for a few hours when the doctor came in.

"We couldn't find anything. We're giving you a shot of Methotrexate in case it was hiding in there somewhere. You have endometriosis lesions as well."

They didn't remove the endometriosis but said they'd be happy to perform another surgery in a few months to remove it if I wanted.

I had the shot of Methotrexate. It's a cancer drug that stops cells from multiplying and causes nausea, vomiting, diarrhoea, abdominal pain ... and you can't get pregnant for at least three months while it's still in your system. It can make you more vulnerable to infection and cause temporary abnormalities in liver function.

I was put in the maternity ward for my recovery. My husband stayed with me. Across the hall was a couple with a beautiful baby girl. Why do they put someone who's just gone through a pregnancy loss on a maternity ward? It's so insensitive.

That night when one of the nurses helped me up to go to the bathroom, I fainted. I came round with doctors and nurses all around me and a blood pressure reading of around 60/40. They were frantically trying to get a second IV in. My blood pressure recovered and I stopped the meds to avoid another episode.

The next morning the hospital photographer came by to ask if we wanted a picture of our baby.

A nurse asked if I wanted to leave right away or wait until the afternoon to see the doctor again. Given my fainting the previous night, we decided to wait until the afternoon to make sure I could walk without passing out, and to see the doctor again; who showed up in the late afternoon.

"So, we finally got those hCG results. They were zero. You weren't pregnant anymore."

"So," I said, after a pause, "there wasn't an ectopic?"

"No," she said, shifting in her seat.

"And the bleeding," I said, "that you saw on the ultrasound? Probably just the extra blood from the pregnancy?"

"Yes," she said. "Probably."

"When can I go home?"

I can still recall the disdain in her eyes as she said, "Honestly, most people would have already left. I don't know why you're still here."

Eight months later, I finally saw a specialist who ran tests and recommended IVF (in-vitro fertilization) and freezing my eggs. We stalled and a few months later when we went back, my FSH (follicle stimulating hormone) had shot up to thirty-four – too high to be allowed IVF. I was diagnosed with diminished ovarian reserve, endometriosis, and single MTHFR mutation. MTHFR is a gene that contains instructions for making an enzyme that's important for metabolising folate (also known as folic acid or vitamin B9).

When I finally hit that point – what I call my 'fertility rock bottom,' I received incredible motivation to heal myself and completely commit to my journey.*

It only took two and a half months of sticking to a strict fertility diet*, cleansing our house* and personal care routines of toxins, and committing to a daily fertility mind-body practice,* and I was finally pregnant. Naturally, the old-fashioned way. I now have a beautiful sixteen-month-old boy who fills our hearts with joy.

I know I still have 'infertility' but I truly believe that when I stop nursing, whenever that may be, and I completely commit to my baby journey again, I will be blessed with another child. No matter what pain and loss you've experienced, I hope you can find the strength to believe in miracles and know that you can be a mommy or a daddy if that's what you want. No one can stop you, except you.

*Please visit my website for more details

Anna Rapp @tomakeamommy

(Link to blog: https://www.tomakeamommy.com/my-first-miscarriage/)

Each loss counts

I've been pregnant six times but only one of those lasted full term.

Seeing that pink line on a pregnancy test should fill you with happiness, but after so many disappointments I came to dread a positive result. This may seem crazy considering we were desperately trying for a baby, but after experiencing multiple pregnancy losses, for me, a positive didn't always mean success.

I had three losses at five, six and nine weeks. I also had at least two chemical pregnancies, or early pregnancy losses, where I had positive tests at four weeks, but usually by five weeks it had all gone wrong. These early losses were just as emotionally painful as the ones that happened a little further along.

I was recently asked at a consultation with a fertility clinic how many times I'd been pregnant and how many pregnancy losses I'd had. I answered six and explained details about each. When I explained about the early losses which had each happened around four to five weeks, the consultant said she only wanted to know about any 'confirmed' pregnancies, i.e. the ones that had made it to the six-week scan. This made it feel like the early pregnancy losses didn't count, yet, I felt the heartache of each and every one of them, so to me, they do matter. I'll carry each one of those losses in my heart forever.

A pregnancy loss is the most devastating blow no matter what stage of your pregnancy it occurs. You should be allowed to grieve every loss.

Karen co-founder @fertilitycircle

BABY LOSS

My heart shattered

When your baby dies, a bit of you dies with them. The life you've been imagining, the plans you had, the parenthood you thought you were entering into are gone. Like your baby, they will never be forgotten; echoes of those dreams creep up on you when you least expect it as you try and find whatever your new 'normal' looks like.

My daughter, Ottilie, was stillborn at thirty-nine weeks. After many years of infertility and two attempts at IVF, (invitro fertilisation) we fell pregnant and had a relatively simple pregnancy. We arrived at the hospital to begin the induction process and quickly it became apparent that something was wrong. Nothing good comes from being moved to a side ward. On the third attempt to find a heartbeat it hit me ... the realisation that no one was hitting the emergency button ... it was all too late.

One of the hardest things to cope with is the long list of unanswered questions. So many whys and what-ifs – the never-ending, simple ones: what colour were her eyes, would she have been a good sleeper, would she have looked more like me or her dad? The more destructive, difficult ones: what if I'd been induced earlier, why didn't I know, could I have done anything differently? Coming to terms with never knowing the answer to any of them is a long road, and one I suspect I may never finish walking.

Every experience of baby loss is different, unique situations and personal stories, but some things that I've found useful I've shared below.

You might be locked into your own experience but seeking out the solace of people who truly understand is a tonic like no other. When you're ready, many are willing to share their stories through Instagram or support groups. Talking to someone anonymously or in person, who truly understands, enables you to express your feelings in a way you may not realise you need, until it presents itself.

Making plans doesn't mean you have to stick to them. We made some big decisions to keep plans we'd made before Ottilie was born and also made new ones. Allowing ourselves the choice to back out at any stage and permitting ourselves to walk away has meant we've seen everything through. The pressure of feeling like you have to be present when your heart is hurting and your mind can't focus, is suffocating. Understanding that has been perhaps the greatest tool in our survival kit.

Talking helps more than you can imagine. My husband and I find it easiest to talk outside, walking side by side. Fresh air and nature often take the edge off emotional or difficult conversations. Counselling has been useful for us both, helping to shape our thoughts and understand our feelings; but come to it in your own time. Talking about Ottilie will never fail to bring me joy; not the joy I expected as a parent, but hearing her name will always be special.

The truth about stillbirth is that it hurts like nothing I've ever known. I didn't expect the physical pain; long after the stitches had healed, the tightness in my chest remains. A deep, drawing, suffocating pain that can wash over me again in an instant ... but thankfully, that doesn't happen so often now. My heart was shattered, I was scrabbling around to try and put the pieces back together. As time moves forward the pieces take a new form, not in the same order, and there will always be a hole left by her absence, but I'm learning to live with it.

Katie Ingram @withoutottilie

From one baby loss dad to another

I'm sorry you're reading this. It sucks that you're here. You're not alone. I'm a father to three pregnancy losses and a stillborn daughter named Joy. I'm also a dad to an energetic five-year-old son and a rainbow new-born daughter.

It's natural to feel heartbroken, overwhelmed, disappointed and hurt. It's also natural to feel nothing at all. I remember feeling sadness, disappointment and concern for my wife when we had our pregnancy losses. They were one after another over eighteen months. The hurt was present but manageable, so I never addressed it. I didn't share our losses with family or friends until after our third loss. Looking back, I wish I'd told them about our struggles earlier. It would've taken away the stress of keeping the secret, and their love and support would've helped. The story of our journey might also have been helpful to loved ones who were perhaps going through something similar. Quietly. In pain. Just like us.

I thought we'd finally passed the hurdle. Our string of bad luck with our three pregnancy losses was over. We were having a daughter. Everything was perfect. Everything was fine. Until it wasn't. No heartbeat. Our daughter was stillborn. She had ten fingers and ten toes. She had lips just like mine. We left the hospital without our child. I was destroyed.

In the early part of my grief I'd spend every night in the basement alone, crying. I'd listen to music that would make me cry. It helped. I could let the pain out through my tears. You don't have to be strong if you're not feeling strong. Cry. Breakdown.

I was searching for answers. I'd spend hours each night Googling, searching for ways to help myself heal, trying to find peers and other dads who'd been through the loss of a child. Facebook groups, Instagram hashtags, Reddit forums. I'd read their stories. They shared my pain. They got it.

There are dads out there who are going through a similar loss, right now. Some dads have worked beyond this pain. We're having those difficult conversations. It was helpful to know that I wasn't alone — that sadly, others like me, from all walks of life and every corner of the world, know this hurt. A brotherhood. All of us wounded. Connect with us if you're up to it.

I journaled my feelings, writing out thoughts and emotions I wasn't ready to share with my wife or anyone else. It helped, releasing the built-up tension and grief. It documented our story. My daughter Joy's story. She was real. She was with us. She is remembered. She is loved.

After about three months of searching for answers and working towards a self-directed healing, I began creating a Care Package for dads suffering from pregnancy loss, stillbirth and infant loss. During my healing process, I found a lot of support for moms suffering from loss, but it was much harder to find something designed especially for dads. I'm proud of what I put together and I wish it had existed when I was trying to understand my own grief. It's not a magic pill, but I wanted to give dads a starting point for healing. So far, the Care Package has helped hundreds of dads and families suffering from pregnancy loss, stillbirth and infant loss.

I also shared our stillbirth story on Instagram. It was so healing to share. I was scared at first to put our story out into the world, but I was blown away by all the love and support from the child loss community. Dads. Moms. Families. Again, you're not alone. Whatever you're feeling it's natural. We're all different and we all feel the loss differently.

Nearly two years later, the hurt comes and goes. Having our rainbow daughter hasn't made the pain of losing Joy any easier. My relationship with my stillborn daughter remains strong and continues to evolve. I still think about her every day. I talk to her and some days I write to her. My love for her is real. You might feel the same way, you might not. However you feel, it's okay. There's no right. There's no wrong.

Share your pain through journaling your thoughts and emotions, or if you're ready, share with your partner. Your pain needs an outlet. Build your community in real life or online of dads, moms and families who are more seasoned in their grief. It helps. And when you're ready, if you feel up to it, be helpful to others. It helps you move forward more than you'll ever believe.

With that, if you feel I can be of service to you, please reach out. I'm here.

Sending love,

Gabriel Soh @lovecommadad

One year on: A letter to my younger self

I see you, bereaved mother. I see you lying there, shell-shocked and numb, having just given birth to your dead baby. I see you struggling to breathe, struggling to feel, struggling to know what life is going to be like.

Let me tell you this, straight up. The next year will be the hardest of your life. You will shed more tears than you thought possible. You will hit the lowest point of your life, and find yourself in the deepest, darkest, blackest hole.

There will be times you wonder if you can survive this.

There will be times you wonder if you would like to survive this.

You will feel rage – a deep, burning, uncontrollable anger – at the world, at fate, at yourself. You will feel envy, jealousy, despair and fear. You will hurt inside – a physical pain, and you will curl up and embrace it, whilst also begging for it to go away.

There will be times you lie on the sofa, hugging your daughter's ashes, trying to pretend that they're a living, breathing baby.

There will be times you lie on the floor, unable to get up as the weight in your chest drags you down.

So, what hope can I offer?

Just this.

There is no end to the darkness, but slowly, light will come back into your life.

You will learn to breathe again.

You will learn to live again.

You will learn to hope again.

They say that motherhood changes you, and it does – in ways you could never imagine. The hardship and pain you suffer will cause you to look inside yourself and take the first step on a long journey of discovery. You will learn so much about yourself in this first year – your fears, your dreams, your strengths, your weaknesses.

You are a phoenix and you will rise from the ashes. This rising will take longer than a day, a week, a month. There won't be a time when you suddenly turn around and think, I am whole again. A small part of you will always feel incomplete. But you will learn to embrace that void inside you for what it is – the child you hold in your heart.

And even though the grief may crash over you like a wave pounding the sand, driving you to your knees, you will be ready for it, and embrace it, because it's not something bad, to be choked back or pushed down, but a manifestation of a wild, everlasting, beautiful love. A love that will last as long as you live.

After death comes new life.

Out of pain and heartbreak comes strength.

Strength does not lie in being stoic. It's not putting on a brave face and pretending to the world that everything is okay, while deep inside, you battle to keep down the feelings that swirl in your belly and claw at your throat. Strength is accepting these feelings, seeking to understand them and the deeper feelings that lie beneath them, then learning to let go of them.

One year on, I am still on this road of discovery. Some days are harder than others. I am not strong yet, but I am stronger.

It's still hard for me to think of her and be happy rather than sad. But that's okay. Grief is love and I choose love over emptiness.

So, when the days are at their darkest, cling to hope.

You will survive.

You will learn to live again.

And you will always be a mother.

Alison @footprintsonourhearts @alisoningleby

Pregnancy and infant loss awareness day

Taken from an Instagram post from 15 October 2019

There are so many emotions that a woman feels when they see a positive pregnancy test. Some dream about seeing two lines for years and years. Some finally do get to see that positive result and are in disbelief, so they spend more money testing to make it seem real. Finally, they believe the test result.

The heart-breaking reality is that the emotional adrenaline rush can be taken away in an instant. Hearing the gut-wrenching words: "There's no heartbeat," is by far the worst experience ever!

For some women, they carry their sweet babies to full-term only to lose them. A distressing event for any mother to go through.

October 15th is #pregnancyandinfantlossawarenessday. I love that awareness is being spread and the silence is being broken. It's real, and it happens more than we realize.

We must be mindful of asking our dear friends when are they going to 'try again' or when is it 'time for the next one' comments. You never know their personal struggle! Maybe they are trying and it's been years of no luck. Maybe after trying for a long time they just recently lost a baby, and your comment cuts to the core and reminds them of their pain all over again. I pray that as people we can be more sensitive and aware of this struggle.

I pray for you who have angels in heaven. I pray that you can have a chance to be a mom someday. I'm thankful for my struggle so I can be there for you. I'm thankful for all the women I've met through this journey. I'm a better person because of it.

I have a necklace that I cherish that has the birthstones of each of us in our family. The diamond stone in the middle is to honor my thirteen lost babies. What item do you have to help you honor your babies that you cherish and love?

Thinking of you today and know my heart is with you as we honor all the babies who left us too soon. You are not forgotten. Your babies are not forgotten. You aren't alone!

Karmann Wennerlind @karmannwennerlind

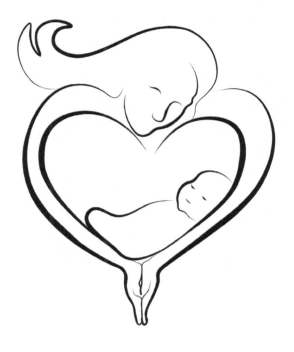

You carry your baby in your heart

Esme's story

My pregnancy with my first baby was largely problem-free. The thrill I felt at seeing the 'positive' result pop up on the pregnancy test was unreal, and the joy I experienced preparing to welcome my baby was the greatest I'd ever known. Our excitement was shared by so many of our family and friends, and we couldn't wait to meet the first little Brunker. I devoured every pregnancy book going, and had already started on the baby manuals. I attended NCT (National Childbirth Trust) and NHS (National Health Service) antenatal classes. I thought I was doing all I could to give my baby the best chance. I don't think I took it for granted that a positive pregnancy test guarantees a healthy living baby at the end of it, but I celebrated every milestone reached as getting closer to the ultimate prize.

Seeing our perfect-looking little creation 'jumping around' on the screen during our twelve-week scan was such a thrilling moment, and our baby became known as 'the bean'. The anomaly scan went well, and then it seemed no time at all before we reached twenty-four weeks – sometimes known as viability – and with every passing week, my confidence grew along with my belly that all was well, and we eagerly awaited the arrival of our first baby just like many other expectant parents. I passed all the checks with flying colours at every midwife appointment. Had I felt the baby move? Yes! Our magic little bean would often be doing somersaults inside of me. I imagined I was growing a future Olympian. Any swollen ankles? Nope. Headaches occasionally, and one migraine, but apart from that no issues, and I knew to report any headaches that lasted an unusually long time or caused visual disturbances.

My midwife would comment according to the progress of my growing bump and the speed of the baby's heartbeat whether she thought I was having a boy or a girl. I found it so funny that her prediction would change each time. One week when I said that the baby had been a bit quieter than normal, she remarked that I must have been busy that day and not noticed the movements so much. When I corrected her that I'd actually been relaxing most of that day, hence noticing that the baby wasn't moving as much, she repeated her claim that I'd probably just been too preoccupied, and said I could go to hospital to be checked if I was ever worried about movements … but if I did that more than a couple of times, I would no longer be eligible to give birth on the midwife-led birthing unit as I'd outlined in my birth plan. As if that was the worst thing that could happen.

I didn't think anything more of it – the baby had gone back to its full regular gymnastic routines, so I presumed that wouldn't be necessary. When we passed the much-fêted 'full term' of thirty-seven weeks, we felt we were on the home straight – what could possibly go wrong? Our hospital bags were packed, the nursery beautifully decorated, the brand-new buggy, painstakingly chosen from a dizzying array of options, was unpacked and waiting. All that remained was for me to face up to the final hurdle of giving birth. I'm ashamed to now admit that, at that point, all I could focus on was that I was terrified of the pain of labour.

And then at thirty-eight weeks and two days our world as we knew it changed forever. I awoke feeling tired. We'd had a disturbed night as a picture had fallen off the wall in the nursery in the early hours of the morning with a huge crash, and our outside light in the garden had turned on almost simultaneously, making us wonder if we were being burgled. A peek through our curtains reassured us when we saw a hedgehog snuffling around on our decking, and when everything else in the house seemed quiet, we went back to sleep.

My PE teacher husband had a morning of coaching to embark upon - introducing his new cohort of year seven boys to rugby, while I was glad to be able to head back to bed. I will forever hate myself for falling asleep while propped up in bed reading. I awoke having napped on my back that morning. When Mark returned home, he asked how the baby was. I replied that I didn't recall any movements all morning. The last I remembered was when I bounced away on my birthing ball watching TV the previous evening, and when I thought about it, the baby had been unusually quiet again the whole of the previous day – hence me remembering that final kick so clearly. I think part of me was relieved to feel that reassurance after a day of not experiencing many kicks or wriggles. I was then racking my brain as to whether they'd been moving normally that whole week and was horrified to realise that I simply didn't know. I obviously hadn't been paying enough attention.

We tried the tricks we'd heard were sure to get the baby moving. I drank cold orange juice, lay on my side. Nothing. We rang the labour ward and they advised us to try what we had already. We explained that we'd done that, and the baby still hadn't moved. They told us to come in to be checked over. We felt a little nervous, unsure of what this could mean. We took our things in, including the baby's car seat, just in case we had to be whisked in for an emergency c-section. That was the worst-case scenario in our minds at that point.

The car journey to the hospital was silent. I don't think we even had the radio on as I concentrated on my very quiet womb, and Mark no doubt with his mind racing yet trying to drive calmly and not panic. We were kept outside of the door to the maternity assessment unit for what felt like an eternity on arrival. I remember being eager to find out what was happening when we did head in, but still no thoughts of it being too serious at this stage.

The midwife was a little brusque as she asked where our straps for the machine that monitors the baby's heartbeat and movements were – she assumed we'd been in for monitoring before. We had to explain that this was our first time coming in for a check over. Her manner did soften slightly as she found a new set for us and said they would be ours to keep in case we needed to return at any point, but her voice changed as she ran the Doppler wand over my tummy, searching for the baby's heartbeat. She was softly murmuring that she couldn't find it, but that she could be wrong. She said that she'd be back as soon as possible with a doctor.

I remember looking up at Mark searching his face for answers, for reassurance, and I could tell he was barely holding back tears, trying to be strong for the both of us as we waited to hear what would be the worst news of our lives. I couldn't believe what was happening as the ultrasound machine that was wheeled in brought nothing but more silence as two young-looking doctors muttered to each other. Mark had tears streaming down his face at this point and I just wanted to scream at them, "What's happening, why aren't you talking to us?" I don't think my brain would accept the seriousness of our situation. I felt angry, scared, and confused more than anything. But instead of speaking, all I could utter was the most animal-like howl of despair upon hearing the words: "I'm sorry, your baby has died."

What happened next was more like an out-of-body experience – that's certainly how I remember it looking back anyway - as if detaching from that most unspeakable pain and horror was the only way I could cope. In my memories, I'm an observer watching my world crumble in front of me; I'm being shoved violently off a cliff edge as I plummet into a dark chasm with no chance of rescue. I know that at some point I was led out of the cubicle, sobbing uncontrollably and barely able to put one foot in front of the other, but I recall thinking to myself, "I need to be kept away from the other mums in here. This must be horrible to listen to." I still wonder whether the woman being monitored in the next cubicle who heard everything ever thinks about us.

After we'd endured a further ultrasound to confirm that our baby was definitely dead, we were taken through to the hospital's bereavement suite, the Star Room. It reminded me of a Travelodge hotel room, complete with kettle and a mini-fridge. None of it seemed real. The midwife who first came to speak to us in there sat down next to me on the sofa with tears in her eyes. She spoke to us calmly and gently. I can't remember her full name but there was the name Angel on her name badge and I thought how apt it was. She said how sorry she was and answered my questions about the next steps. My heart sank at hearing how long the induction process might take because my body showed no signs of being in labour at that time. Neither my brain nor my body wanted to believe this was really happening.

I wanted everything to be over fast but resisted Mark's suggestion that I should have a c-section. I couldn't bear the thought that my baby would be surgically removed from me like some kind of tumour. I had never had any surgery in my life and knew that it was a major operation - one that I'd be more than willing to endure if it meant the chance of a living baby at the end of it, but not under these circumstances. I wanted to do our little bean the honour of at least delivering them the way we'd planned, to know that I'd been able to do that last act for them and for me. I know many bereaved mothers have the opposite response, and cannot fathom how cruel it is to go through labour with no hope of any happy ending after all that emotional and physical stress. But I almost welcomed the prospect of labour as something to focus on rather than the reality we were dealing with.

Mark had the unenviable task of breaking the news to our parents over the phone. I truly don't know how he found the strength or the words to have those conversations, and I know their cries of disbelief and despair will forever haunt him. After I'd been given a pessary to prepare my cervix, we were given a 'Sands' (Stillbirth and neonatal death society), bereavement support pack to take home and digest before we returned to the hospital the following evening for induction.

We didn't get a lot of rest that night, for obvious reasons, and we hadn't yet told all of our family and friends what was happening. We needed time and space to come to terms with the news and I couldn't face all of the messages of sympathy, fearing they would make what was happening all the more real.

We went for a walk in the early hours of the morning and chose a name for our baby: Esme for a girl, Toby for a boy. I was induced as planned on Sunday evening and after a mercifully quick labour with little pain relief, managed to deliver naturally at 5.39 am on Monday 23rd September. We had a little girl: Esme.

There was no obvious reason why she'd died as my placenta appeared completely normal. And Esme was perfectly formed – a healthy 7lb 1oz weight and 55cm length. We spent time making memories with her in the Star Room, including taking some photographs, but to me it was painfully obvious that she'd already gone – the condition of her body quickly deteriorating, (very upsetting for us), being a brutal reminder of that fact, though she was still beautiful to us.

I was not of the belief that the damage to her skin was evidence of her having suffered in the womb and that it was likely caused from the time she was inside me after she'd died, and then passing through my birth canal. But everything was so far removed from how I imagined we would spend time with our baby after they were born, that I didn't want to linger in that room for too long.

It would never be easy to say goodbye and I didn't want my memories of her to be tarnished by how she looked towards the end of our time with her. Some of our family came to meet her, and I'm forever grateful that they were brave enough to do so. I wish I'd granted them their wish to hold her, but I worried that the blankets she was swaddled in would come loose and that they'd be alarmed, or even horrified by what they saw, or say something that would upset me. I wanted to protect her from anything less than the pure adoration she deserved.

Esme's post-mortem results were available to us on the 4th November – exactly six weeks after she'd been born. The consultant who spoke to us about them was only able to confirm that she was perfect, as was my placenta, so no cause of death had been found, and to this day we are none the wiser why she died. Although of course, I have since invented a million and one reasons why it was all my fault.

We told our consultant and bereavement midwife that my antenatal care could have been better in hindsight, as although all the checkboxes were ticked during my appointments – blood pressure taken, urine tested, bump measured, etc, I was never told why it was so important to carry out all those checks, and why pregnant mothers need to monitor foetal movements, as stillbirth was never an issue that I was made aware of. I'm conscious how midwives must be reluctant to scare expectant mothers and don't want them worrying unnecessarily, but it was agreed in our post-mortem results appointment that more information could have been given to highlight warning signs. We should all know how and why to seek help if any alarming symptoms appear during pregnancy, and have medical professionals willing to act quickly if a baby requires assistance.

Sadly, I had no instinct that anything was wrong with Esme, and I will never forgive myself for not monitoring her movements more carefully, but many bereaved mothers do report that they didn't feel quite right before they found out that their baby had died, or that they'd noticed a change in their baby's pattern of movements.

My experience with Esme has taught me that it's crucial to listen to a pregnant woman's instinct, and a midwife should be happy to discuss any worries and act upon them when necessary. Don't rely on advice from family members, friends or even the internet. If you feel that a midwife isn't listening, you can ask to speak to another member of the team. If you're still anxious that you're not being heard, contact the day assessment unit within the maternity unit or seek advice from the Consultant Midwife. Sadly, even the professionals can get it wrong, and no one knows your body and your baby better than you do.

Since Esme died, I've been involved in attempts to improve maternity/bereavement care and hopefully prevent stillbirths in the first place, by participating in a local Maternity Services Liaison Committee at the hospital where I gave birth. I'm a parent speaker at 'Sands' Improving Bereavement Care Study Days and have undertaken training to be a Befriender for my local 'Sands' group. I've also been inspired to write a beautifully illustrated book for families affected by the death of a baby. Many people who experience this type of loss have already included children, siblings, cousins, even family friends in preparation to welcome a new baby into their family, so it can be a distressing time for children affected by a bereavement of this kind. Even if they don't grieve in the way that the adults around them might, they'll almost certainly be aware that the grownups around them are shocked and sad.

Although Esme was our first baby, we had young children in our family who needed to be told the tragic news, and it was challenging to know how to guide them through what was a confusing and upsetting time. My instinct was to turn to a picture book to help, but I struggled to find one suitable. I wanted straightforward, honest language and imagery that would reflect our situation and beliefs, but most of what was available back then just didn't feel 'right' or good enough. So, I decided to write and publish my own. I was lucky to connect with an incredibly talented and generous illustrator, Gillian Gamble, who supported my dream and helped bring These Precious Little People to life. It's a creation that we're so proud of. We know that in the time since its publication in December 2018, it has already helped bring comfort to thousands of families so far. It's been designed so that anyone can use this book as a positive focus during times of grief - to bring comfort, but also help them remember a precious part of their family with love and pride.

My nephews, niece, young cousin, and my two children born after Esme died, all know about the little girl that made me a mummy. We visit her grave, we have plants at home in her memory, and we perform acts of kindness in her honour. She's very much part of our lives still. They ask me questions about her; we speak her name and we all miss her and wish she was here. *These Precious Little People* is inspired by them and the desire we share to keep our connection to Esme alive. It lets them know that it's OK to talk about her.

My hope has always been that *These Precious Little People* will help other families who've been searching for a bereavement support resource for children, that they feel helps tell the story of their baby, and acknowledges the pain felt by them. *These Precious Little People* can be read in the immediate aftermath of devastating news, or months or years later. It can be used by the family as a framework to have open and honest conversations, explaining that the grief they are experiencing (or witnessing), is normal and healthy. It doesn't claim to provide all the answers - for how can there ever be any good reason why a much-loved baby dies, but it does offer support and understanding, and suggests ways that families can pay tribute to their little ones gone too soon. I used simple language that avoids the euphemisms often associated with death that can be ambiguous, and at times unnecessarily frightening for children. The text is written in poetic verse so that it flows well for adults reading it with their children, who can follow the rhythm present on the pages but, equally, time can be taken to linger over the stunning and vibrant artwork. Gillian's illustrations befit the seriousness and importance of this subject and lend a sensitive beauty that will appeal to both children and adults. It has a timeless feel and reflects the varied range of baby-loss experiences. It was important to us that all families, regardless as to their ethnicity, religious beliefs or culture, could relate to the book, appreciate the artwork and draw comfort from the words.

All proceeds from sales of the book go to Joel The Complete Package, a small Midlands-based charity that supports families affected by the death of a baby during pregnancy or soon after birth, including those parenting after loss.

Frankie Brunker @thesepreciouslittlepeople

We never forget

Imagine being told, "In a couple of hours, everything you thought you knew about life will be gone. Your whole belief system and soul will be ripped out of you. You'll experience indescribable loss, yet somehow, you'll get through it."

Baby loss is multi-faceted, complex and messy. The pain is indescribable. The moment I heard those words, "There's no heartbeat," nothing seemed real.

What it feels like to lose a baby

Your worst nightmares seem like daydreams; reality is too much to bear. How can you move on with your life when all you see is your baby, the memories and trauma replaying over and over? Separate to the physical pain of your baby being taken, your core is ripped out of you and nothing is as it once was. Even society treats you as an outsider.

Instant connections

It's not a club I ever wanted to join, but it's an amazing place to be. When you meet another mum whose experienced loss, you don't even need to speak. There's an instant connection, an unspoken mutual understanding. You build resilience over time and survive, because you know others have endured this before you and lived to tell the tale. They are living proof that life goes on, that we can recover from this catastrophic blow to our lives.

"In baby loss, we accept, we adjust, but we never forget."

Still a mama

All your life philosophies and parenting approaches fly out the window when a baby dies. Your entire being is deconstructed in ways you never knew possible. It's unimaginable that anyone can survive the aftermath. Living on without your child is unthinkable; continuing to function seems impossible. But what I learned is that just because your baby isn't there, doesn't mean you're not a mother – you will continue to parent your child every day, just not in the way you'd hoped or planned.

"I am and always will be 'Still a Mama' to Gracie Rose, stillborn on 7 July 2016: always loved, never forgotten."

The most agony, the most love

Losing Gracie meant everything had changed, but even in the extreme pain of loss, the destruction of everything you thought you knew is liberating. There's strength in being vulnerable. It takes bravery to be open to the hurt, to let it matter. This remarkable loss is the most agony I've ever felt, yet it holds the most love I've ever known. It's also given me a new definition of self, a new way of seeing, and a new love – one so strong that it made saying "hello" and "goodbye" in the same day worth all the pain.

What I've learned along the way

- Just breathing is ENOUGH.

- Don't let suffering be a measure of your love. Oh, how I punished myself in those early days. Relief from grief is allowed; punishing yourself isn't helpful.

- Your mental health is a priority, self-care is a priority, your existence is a priority.

- You're still a kind person with a good heart if you say "no". Don't expect yourself to be the person you were before; this is a new you, and you'll be getting to know yourself for the next few years. On that note, don't give yourself timescales to feel better, particularly in the early months. I did and set myself up for the biggest fall of my life.

- You'll lose some of your support network. This is normal in baby loss. People will do things that hurt, and it's okay to take a year out and reassess relationships and friendships. It's okay to distance yourself from people who are pregnant, to unfollow people on social media.

You're not a bad person for doing this.

- It's helpful to speak with another baby-loss mum. It confirms that your irrational thoughts are very normal. You'll bond over your shared experiences of how you can deal with this tragedy.

- Motherhood seems like some cruel joke. There are reminders everywhere. Protect yourself as much as you need to. Be aware that grief stings when you least expect it. Don't fight it. It will always win.

- Your relationship with your partner will be tested beyond belief.

- Live each day in honour of your baby. They are never more than a thought away. You'll learn a new kind of love that can only be experienced to be understood.

- Live minute by minute, hour by hour, and day by day when you can.

Lisa Sharrock @stillamama

I blamed myself for my stillbirth and pregnancy loss

I was born in Colombia, South America, and at the age of thirty-two, I discovered my fallopian tubes were blocked due to severe endometriosis. Even after doing a laparoscopy to try and unblock them, it didn't work, making IVF (in vitro fertilization) the only option. My husband was supportive; however, the emotional stress was heavy on both of us. My first cycle was successful – they retrieved thirty-four eggs and fourteen of them fertilized. I had four embryos transferred and I had a daughter who is now fourteen-years-old.

In 2009, we decided to have a second baby. We weren't worried as our first IVF cycle had been so successful. Secretly, we both desperately wanted a son this time. We started our next cycle, but due to a mistake in the medication dosage made by the clinic, I got OHSS (ovarian hyperstimulation syndrome – where far too many follicles grow), and my cycle was cancelled. The RE (reproductive endocrinologist) offered us another cycle at no cost.

On my next IVF cycle, we got four embryos, one of which was less developed, but the clinic said we could transfer all four. We made up our minds that the three well-developed embryos were male – they had to be, didn't they? We got a positive pregnancy test and were convinced we were expecting a boy. We decided to find out the sex of the baby at the scan and to our surprise, it was a girl! We hadn't expected that and it took us a few days to accept.

I had a good pregnancy, everything was normal, but no one knew I was developing a blood issue. At thirty-nine weeks, three days before my due date, our baby girl, Isabelle, died in my womb due to a blood clot in the umbilical cord – but I still had to deliver her. Devastated and lost, I felt guilty for what happened, believing it was because I wanted a boy, not a girl.

We pursued a fourth round of IVF less than two months later.

Again, I got a positive test, but I lost my baby at seven weeks. I blamed it on my sadness at the loss of Isabelle, the stress and fear combined with other personal issues.

In 2011, my husband and I felt completely lost and didn't know what our future looked like. Driven by fear and ego, we almost got divorced but chose instead to make some positive changes and stay together.

In 2012, we decided to do our fifth and final round of IVF. This cycle was an amazing experience for us both ... full of love, healthy dialogue and peace, which was a direct result of our internal struggles and the shifts we made together as a team. This last round of IVF thankfully resulted in the birth of our second daughter, who is now seven years old.

Monica Bivas @monicabivas

RESOURCES

Alison Ingleby is an author, podcaster and writer. After her first child, her daughter Skye was stillborn in 2019, she started Footprints on our Hearts, a podcast about baby loss, legacy and learning to live again. The podcast aims to raise awareness of all forms of baby loss and help bereaved parents feel less alone.

If you would like to connect with Alison:
Instagram @footprintsonourhearts @alisoningleby
Twitter @skyesfootprints @aringleby
Footprints on our Hearts podcast is available on your favourite podcast app or on the website: www.footprintsonourhearts.com

Alex is a blogger at Every Body Matters, which is a collection of resources for people who are struggling with infertility, and for those who want to offer their support. The community is very active on Instagram where it raises awareness and offers support for infertility and pregnancy loss.

If you would like to connect with Alex:
Instagram @wheneverybodymatters
Website www.wheneverybodymatters.com
Email hello@wheneverybodymatters.com

Anna Rapp beat the odds and got pregnant naturally after the doctors said it wasn't possible. She blogs at the website 'To Make a Mommy' about how she did it, and encourages her readers to empower themselves and take charge of their fertility journey. She is passionate about clean, green, and healthy living, and shares tips on how to eliminate fertility-harming toxins from your lifestyle, eat a clean, organic, whole-foods diet, and develop a daily mind-body practice for fertility. Anna lives with her husband and two miracles in Virginia.

If you would like to connect with Anna:
Instagram @tomakeamommy

Website https://www.tomakeamommy.com
Facebook https://www.facebook.com/tomakeamommy
Twitter https://twitter.com/tomakeamommy
Pinterest https://www.pinterest.com/tomakeamommy/

Arden Cartrette is a blogger based out of Pittsboro, North Carolina, USA. She started blogging and sharing her fertility journey through social media in 2018, after struggling to get pregnant in her early 20s. After over two and a half years of trying to conceive and suffering two pregnancy losses, Arden and her husband, Kerry, welcomed their double rainbow, Cameron, in February 2020. Since the birth of Cameron, she's continued to share the joys and stresses of motherhood after infertility and pregnancy loss.

If you would like to connect with Arden:
Instagram @ardenmcartrette
Website www.hello-warrior.com

Cat Strawbridge had a seven-year infertility journey, that included IUI, IVF, ICSI and two pregnancy losses. On her fourth IVF cycle, she got pregnant with twins, but sadly lost one of the identical twins at ten weeks. She is all too familiar with the anxiety and stress of baby loss and being pregnant after infertility, which is why she hosts The Finally Pregnant podcast. She is active on her personal Instagram account @tryingyears and is the 'Cat' half of Instagram account @itscatandalice, (the 'Alice' half is @thisisalicerose). Amongst other things, Cat and Alice host Live Your Life: Fertility events – which include talks by health and wellbeing experts and people talking about their own fertility experiences. This offers the opportunity to connect with others who have similar situations to your own, plus there are goody bags and much more. Check out www.catandalice.com which has a global TTC meet up calendar as well as details of upcoming events.

If you would like to connect with Cat:
Instagram @tryingyears
Website www.catstrawbridge.com

Erin Bulcao is thirty-five years old and originally from Mexico City but now lives in Encinitas CA. She has twin eight-and-a-half-year-old girls conceived through IUI, who are her world but who also test her daily. She's a certified yoga teacher and was teaching at Core Power Yoga, but has taken a break whilst going through IVF for the last two-and-a-half years. She's obsessed with NYC and travels there a few times a year because she loves it so much. She met her husband when she was twenty-two, outside a bar and has been married for ten years! She recently started a blog which has helped her tremendously, and hopes it's also helped others either going through infertility, and those wanting to learn more. She's a 'snacker', could eat dessert all day, is a Bravo TV junkie and always has a bowl of cereal before bed.

If you would like to connect with Erin:
Instagram @mybeautifulblunder
Blog www.mybeautifulblunder.com

Frankie Brunker is an author and, since her daughter Esme died, has been involved in attempts to improve maternity/bereavement care (and hopefully prevent stillbirths in the first place), by participating in a local Maternity Services Liaison Committee at the hospital where Esme was born. She's also a parent speaker at Sands Improving Bereavement Care Study Days and has undertaken training to be a Befriender for her local Sands group. She has written and published *These Precious Little People*, a beautifully illustrated book for families affected by the death of a baby.

If you would like to connect with Frankie:
Instagram @thesepreciouslittlepeople
Website links https://preciouslittlepeople.wixsite.com/preciouslittlepeople and http://www.joeltcp.org

Gabriel Soh is father to a stillborn daughter named Joy. He and his wife also experienced three pregnany losses. After Joy's birth, he put together a Care Package; an online, video-based resource as a starting point to help in the healing process for other baby and child loss dads, moms and families. It has helped hundreds start to process, discuss, and understand the grief of pregnancy loss, stillbirth and infant loss.

If you would like to connect with Gabriel:
Website www.lovecommadad.com

Helena Tubridy MA RN RM is a midwife, hypnotherapist, certified fertility coach, mental health counsellor and EMDR therapist. She believes that mindset is key for women and men to optimise natural fertility, and to prepare for IVF success. With a research-based focus, she also combines lifestyle and nutrition with medically accurate information to reduce your time to pregnancy. She feels privileged to help clients with EMDR after pregnancy loss, fatal foetal abnormality, stillbirth and birth trauma. Based in beautiful wild Ireland, Helena works globally via Zoom. Probably due to that accent, her powerful guided meditation audios have received accolades! Her new online course 'Fully Charged Fertility' is out June2020. As a passionate voice for fertility health, Helena is a popular contributor on TV, radio, press and podcast.

If you would like to connect with Helena:
Instagram @helenatubridy
Blogs and commentary https://www.helenatubridy.com

Jackie Figueras, MSN-Ed, RN, CPC, is a passionate and accomplished registered nurse, educator, and fertility support coach. She received her training as a professional certified coach at the Institute for Professional Excellence in Coaching. Her unique combination of being a nurse, an educator, a coach and a patient who struggled with fertility issues, allow her to connect with her clients and provide engaging and interactive programs that set her apart from other communication specialists and fertility coaches. Struggling with fertility issues for years and having four consecutive pregnancy losses, including her daughters' twin, has created a deeper passion for changing healthcare and the fertility journey for many women. She truly understands the impact stress can have on your physical, mental and emotional health and is dedicated to helping guide women on their own journeys to find more balance and peace.

If you would like to connect with Jackie:
Instagram @jackiefigueras
Email jackie@thesupportivemama.com
Website www.thesupportivemama.com

Jalina King is a writer and creator of 'This Side of If', a blog discussing faith, family, and feelings of motherhood after infertility and loss. She and her husband suffered three years of male factor infertility and five pregnancy losses before becoming parents to their three rainbow baby boys. Unable to find support for the unique joys and challenges of motherhood after infertility, Jalina created 'This Side of If' and co-founded the Motherhood After Infertility Facebook group, as a place for other moms to share and discuss how they are forever affected by their time with infertility, even after becoming mothers. She is passionate about infertility and pregnancy loss awareness.

If you would like to connect with Jalina:
Instagram @thissideofif
Website www.thissideofif.com

Jodi Sky Rogers is a Feminine Healing Coach and author. Her personal experience with PCOS, (polycystic ovarian syndrome), fertility challenges and pregnancy loss over the past seven years inspires her to support women going through similar experiences. She is passionate about creating soulful fertility, mindfulness and TTC (trying to conceive) self-care resources and tools to support women on their fertility journey. She is a fertility blogger for the Conceive IVF Gynaecology & Fertility Hospital's 'Fried Eggs & Slow Swimmers' blog. She is the author of Flowering Within and Wild Essence and Daily Cup of Fertility Calm: Tea Meditations, Inspiration and Self-Care Practices for anxiety relief during the Two Week Wait

If you would like to connect with Jodi:
Instagram @thefertilemoon

Website http://jodiskyrogers.com
Facebook Page https://www.facebook.com/
jodiskyrogersauthor/

Justine Bold has personal experience of infertility as she had a twelve year journey to motherhood, finally becoming a mum to twin boys in her forties. She has written articles on infertility and edited a book entitled: *Integrated Approaches to Infertility, IVF and Recurrent Miscarriage* that was published in 2016. She's also co-written a book on mental health that was published in 2019. She works as a University Lecturer and has research interests in lifestyle and nutrition and their links to health problems, such as endometriosis and polycystic ovarian syndrome.

If you would like to connect with Justine:
Twitter @justineboldfood
Instagram @justinebold
Website https://www.worcester.ac.uk/about/profiles/justine-bold

Karen Hanson and her friend Abi created The Fertility Circle following their own personal struggles. The Fertility Circle App is a place people can turn to for instant access to information and support to help empower them on their fertility journey. You can find expert advice, search for local fertility service providers and also connect with others on social chat walls. Download Fertility Circle from the App Store for Apple and Google Play Store for Android.

If you would like to connect with Karen and Abi:
Instagram @fertilitycircle
Email hello@thefertilitycircle.com
Facebook @fertilitycircle

Karmenn Wennerlind is an infertility warrior, recurrent pregnancy loss survivor, mama to three rainbow miracles and one furbaby

If you would like to connect with Karmenn:
Instagram @karmennwennerlind

Katie Ingram documents her experiences of unexplained infertility and the unexplained stillbirth of her daughter in the hope that, by sharing her story, other families feel more able to speak openly about their own. Ottilie was stillborn in April 2019 and the seemingly silent and utterly shocking statistics surrounding stillbirth led Katie to seek out ways to raise awareness. She has written articles for The Independent and The Evening Standard as well as guest blogs, and continues to seek support and understanding from the Instagram community.

If you would like to connect with Katie:
Instagram @withoutottilie
Website www.withoutottilie.com

Dr Katy Huie Harrison PhD is an author, toddler mom and owner of Undefining Motherhood. She lives in Atlanta with her husband (affectionately known on the internet as 'Husband,'), son (Jack) and dog (Charlotte). She believes our society has historically placed too many expectations on women, defining womanhood and motherhood in a way that is restrictive. Her goal is to shift the paradigm about what it means to be a woman and a mother, giving all women a greater sense of agency over their lives.

If you would like to connect with Katy:
Instagram, Pinterest and Twitter @khuieharrison
Website www.undefiningmotherhood.com
Facebook undefiningmotherhood
LinkedIn khuieharrison

Katy Jenkins is twenty-eight years old and lives with her husband Thomas in Exeter, Devon. They've been trying to conceive for five years and have had natural losses and failed IVF transfers. During their journey they decided to create a sock company called 'The Journey Starts Here' with the hope that their socks bring joy to such an incredibly hard journey. It's also a great way for people to tell their story via social media and to connect with other men and women who understand the struggles of infertility. Katy also treats them as her lucky socks. She finds TTC (trying to conceive) accounts on social media extremely helpful and supportive whilst on her journey.

If you would like to connect with Katy and Thomas:
Instagram @thejstartshere
Website www.thejourneystartshere.co.uk

Lauren Gourley Lauren Gourley is twenty-five and comes from Northern Ireland. She experienced a pregnancy loss in January 2020 and it was heart-breaking. She constantly searched for someone online who she could talk to. She didn't want anyone else to feel as alone as she did, so she decided to start her Instagram page so that she can support others and still get supported herself.

If you would like to connect with Lauren:
Instagram @truths_of_miscarriage

Lisa Sharrock runs the blog 'Still A Mama' which she founded after her daughter Gracie was stillborn. 'Still A Mama' has been created to break the silence of baby loss, honour all babies taken too soon, and to help loss mothers on their journey to building a new normal. It also provides an environment to open up about the tragedy that is parenthood after baby loss, and enables loss parents the opportunity to be proud of their babies and the love they have brought to their lives.

If you would like to connect with Lisa:
Instagram @still_a_mama
Facebook still-a-mama and blog www.stillamama.co.uk

Lucy started 'The Rainbow Running & Yoga Club', and it's a community of women who've experienced baby loss or infertility. They hold regular events across the UK where they meet up and run, walk or practice yoga together, and then enjoy a delicious slice of cake or two! They also hold retreat days and weekends. They've recently started holding online events too, which can be great for those who feel anxious about coming along to one of the events, and also provides a brilliant way to connect all the ladies of the Rainbow Running and Yoga Club, regardless of where they live. She cannot express just how freeing and uplifting it can be to meet a group of women who understand, and who you can just be yourself with. You don't need to be a "runner" or a "yogi" to join them, as every woman is welcome.

If you would like to connect with Lucy:
Instagram @_mother_of_one_
Website www.rainbowrunningclub.co.uk

Monica Bivas went through multiple IVF (invitro fertilization) treatments – including the stillbirth of her second daughter – but was determined to try one last time. This time, however, she decided to approach her treatment with mindfulness and positivity which resulted in the birth of her third daughter. She now helps her tribe consciously direct their IVF experience by managing their emotions, shifting their mindsets, and preparing for the ultimate outcome of treatment – a precious baby. She is a regular contributor to the Huffington Post, and has published The IVF Planner, a journal and guide for women undergoing fertility treatment, and has another book forthcoming about her life-changing experience with IVF treatment. She is married to her amazing Israeli husband, Shai, whom she considers her best friend, and has two daughters and one step-daughter. Although born in Colombia, she is deeply in love with her home in Long Island, New York. When not supporting her IVF tribe, she fully immerses herself in being a hands-on mom, and a must in her life is a weekly date with her husband doing one of her favorite activities: dancing.

If you would like to connect with Monica:
Instagram @monicabivas
Facebook monicabivasIVFcoach
Facebook Group Theivfjourney
Twitter @MonicaBivas
Pinterest @monicabivas
Website www.monicabivas.com
LinkedIn monicabivas

Nicola Salmon is a fat-positive and feminist fertility coach. She advocates for change in how fat women are treated on their fertility journey. She supports fat women, and others with disordered eating, who are struggling to get pregnant, to find peace with their body, find their own version of health and finally escape the yo-yo dieting cycle. For more information download: The Fat Girl's Guide to Getting Pregnant: http://nicolasalmon.co.uk/fat-girls-guide-getting-pregnant/

If you would like to connect with Nicola:
Instagram @fatpositivefertility
Website www.nicolasalmon.co.uk

Nora is now pregnant after four pregnancy losses with 'lucky number five'. She is a Mindset Coach and supports women going through pregnancy loss and pregnancy after loss.

If you would like to connect with Nora:
Instagram @thislimboland

Sharna Southan knows first-hand the feeling of where you are right now. She is a life coach specialising in helping women after pregnancy loss to move through the overwhelming grief, reconnect with themselves and their new identity so they can reignite their love for life again.

If you would like to connect with Sharna:
Instagram @sharnasouthan_coaching
Facebook @sharnasouthancoaching
Website www.sharnasouthan.com

Sophie Martin is a Registered Midwife and infertility and baby loss advocate. Currently navigating the bumpy road of IVF, (invitro fertilisation) whilst also honouring the memory of her twin sons Cecil & Wilfred, after their very premature birth and death. She is dedicated to celebrating the power of women, and acknowledging how important it is to support other women on their journey to motherhood.

If you would like to connect with Sophie:
Instagram @the.infertile.midwife
Blog www.theinfertilemidwife.com

Suzanne Minnis experienced three failed IVF (in vitro fertilisation) cycles and a pregnancy loss after conceiving naturally, that left her devastated and wondering if she would ever become a mum. On their fourth cycle, Suzanne and her husband got their BFP, (positive pregnancy test) and she is now mama to their miracle daughter. She now blogs about fertility, IVF and motherhood.

If you would like to connect with Suzanne:
Instagram @the_baby_gaim
Blog www.thebabygaim.com

Yuen Kwan Li has personal experience after having had two pregnancy losses, and she now runs the Instagram and Facebook pages for London Miscarriage Support Group, who have a monthly meet up in London UK, for men and women who have experienced pregnancy loss. It is run by registered psychotherapist Flora Saxby.

If you would like to connect with Yuen:
Instagram @over40_tryingforababy Miscarriage support group:
Instagram @londonmiscarriagesupport
Facebook London Miscarriage Support Group

Thank you for buying this book

It means a lot to me and the contributors that we are helping and supporting you.

Please would you do one thing to help people in the same community as you? If you found this book helpful, would you spread the word by leaving an honest review on the website that you brought it from, as this helps others to find the book and provides social proof. Alternatively, you can leave a review on my website here: www.mfsbooks.com Please also feel free to review the book on your own social media channels.

I love to hear from readers and receive feedback about the *This is* series, after all, the books are for people on the same journey as you, so please contact me at sheila@mfsbooks.com

I'm very passionate that people who haven't experienced fertility treatments understand how it really is, because then they will be in a better position to offer the best kind of support. If you agree, why don't you gift a copy to a family member or friend, especially if you want them to know what you're going through but can't bring yourself to tell them personally.

If you are a professional working in a fertility clinic, a hospital, Early Pregnancy Unit, maternity ward or in your own practice and would like to offer the paperback or ebook as a patient resource to your clients, please contact me at the above email address for bulk discount information.

If you have a podcast or need guest posts for your website, I am always happy to share my story so that it may help others. Just drop me an email.

Don't forget to check out all the other books in the *This is* series, and my standalone book *My Fertility Book, all the fertility and infertility explanations you will ever need, from A to Z* – please see my website www.mfsbooks.com for more details.

I make a small donation from this sale to an appropriate charity in your country; I do this for all my books.

Wishing you all the very best.

Love Sheila x